Raincoat Diary

Lorrena Bishop

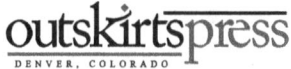

DENVER, COLORADO

Table of Contents

The Introduction

Welcome to my world. It is small, really, with only a few people in it. For years now I have been locked inside my mind with no place to go. With that said, I begin my journey with you. You see, I have a story about fears, sadness, and dreams, everything you have too. Welcome to my diary.

Before I begin, let me introduce myself. My name is Lorrena. I am tempted to say it is something else, but I want you to know me, so yes, that is my real name. I am thirty-eight years old, married, and a mother of two young children, so like many of you, I have a lot to deal with daily. I feel afraid to talk to you, but I will anyway.

As I sit here in my room, only a few words come to mind in describing me: obese, unhappy, and restless. It is the beginning of a new year, and I have all these things inside my mind that I want to accomplish, so I will write them down as proof that I even expressed a desire for change. By the end of this year I want to be 140 pounds thinner, happily employed, and have a new sense of self. My weight is currently 230. I live in Arkansas, where it seems many people—adults and children—are very tall. I know so from comparison to living in other states and towns. The children are very tall for their ages, and I know, because I am a substitute teacher in two elementary schools. I am only four feet, eleven inches tall.. I cannot change my height, so I will not talk of that subject again. I will, however, talk of that which I can change: my weight, financial situation, and mental state.

I have been married for more than eight years. I have a lingering feeling that my husband would rather I kick the bucket than hang around for years and years. I think he regrets marrying me, since I am very cold and distant. I wonder when strangers meet me for the first time if they can tell that I am lonely, but they probably cannot. Strangers are always running around doing their own thing. I doubt that anyone notices others the way we think they do. Sometimes when I look at popular people with twenty best friends, I question if they have any idea what it must be like for those without any friends at all. Walking in someone else's shoes for a while would be an eye opener, some say. I personally would like to get out of my shoes.

If I could describe myself to you, I would say poorly dressed. On any day, I am wearing a T-shirt, old jeans, and raggedy tennis shoes. I have only one pair of shoes. I wear them for everything, from work to playing outside to going to church. I wish I had more shoes. Every dollar my husband makes goes to food or bills. Years have gone by and no money seems to be there for me to spend to look better or feel better. Sometimes I look at women who have nice nails and hair and wonder if they understand what shame I feel for looking so unrespectable. I have the street look. No, not one of a hooker, but one of homeless women with stringy hair and no makeup. I wonder if inside this mind of mine there is hope for a better person. I would love to be so much more improved.

I see acquaintances sometimes, and I can sense they too think of me as fat and badly dressed. I can see it when they look at me, without any words at all. I can just tell, because it cuts like a knife in my heart. How do I describe the look of snobbery or disgust? You have to experience it to understand what I am saying. Through a lifetime of financial struggles, I think I have gotten used to allowing it to be okay to be in public looking so shabby. If the fashion police were to come in to town,

I would surely be the one they chose to take down for fashion crimes. I have stretch pants that make me look horrible.

No one wants to see a fat woman in a raincoat on a sunny day every day of the year. That is who I am, though, a woman in a raincoat. The raincoat is a man's ugly blue jacket with holes in the pockets. I wear it all the time for security. You know how children have a security blanket? Well, the blue raincoat is my pretend world that everything is okay. I use it to cover up fat arms and bad clothes. All the while, everyone is making faces at the bad style and choice of clothing every day of the year, even hot days. Yes, here I am writing about my raincoat. The whole reason for my book *Raincoat Diary* is my hiding from the worst possible enemy I know, which is me. I wish I were not here at the moment complaining about loneliness. I wish I were on the phone with my best friends from high school making weekend getaway plans and laughing about our trips to the beach. I don't have any friends to talk about at this time. I don't sit around crying about that fact, but my heart wants good friends to share secrets with.

What kind of friend would I be? I know I could be a good one who prayed a lot and always listened to problems and helped with life situations. There have been many moments in my life when I wondered why people didn't stay long in my world. I wondered if I had been just a little better to them, would they have stuck around longer. I then realized that people come and go, and there is not much we can do to stop them.

My shame of my body image has taken over all of my thought processes, and I feel that I have nothing to offer others at the moment. What I want is to learn to love me first and then find the best friend ever. She will be kind and good to others and love to exercise. My new best friend will be everything I want to be too. She will be smart and love talking about any subject. She will be a good listener and enjoy a funny movie. If I could choose a new best friend, she would have a heart of gold. She would want to help those in need. She would call me often.

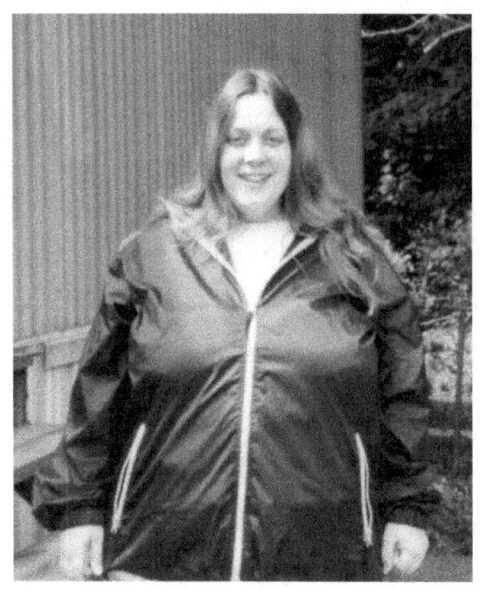

Here I am at my highest weight of 240 in my raincoat in July. It was a hot summer day, and I wore my raincoat anyway. I hoped that no one would notice my fat body if I wore this coat. This photo was taken a very long time ago, when I first started wearing my dear reliable raincoat. Looking at this photo now, I can see that nothing is hidden. It just makes me look silly. Some people accessorize so you don't see fat. I wear a raincoat.

Dear Diary,

January 7, 2009

I went on a diet yesterday. I started exercising today. I only made it ten minutes. Sad, really, the lack of energy I have from being so overweight. I found the perfect show to watch on television last night. The first week one guy lost more than fifteen pounds, and honestly I wondered how I could do that too. What a miracle to lose so much weight in that amount of time! No one can tell me that is safe, but who cares when it's weight loss!

In my quest to better my situation, it occurred to me that I must fix my whole self, not just portions. Last Sunday I started back going to church. Maybe my spiritual side needed recharging. After all, I did feel a need to hit everyone with a bat for no reason. I felt that the sweet me that I once knew died a few years ago.

Church was stressful because everyone was dressed so nicely. I was dressed in pants and an ugly black shirt, and I had no idea that my underpants were showing all during Sunday school. Why did I moon people with my butt? I meant to make new friends, not gross people out. First impressions are everything. I told myself that I was going to church to visit God. Somehow it turned into having a large anxiety attack about my pants showing my butt. Why had I turned religion and visiting God into being about me? Okay, note to self: wear longer shirts to church. I sat in Sunday school staring across the table at a couple. I will call them Matching Duo. She had diamonds on her neck, wrists, and fingers. So did her husband. He had a bright tie that matched her scarf and dress. Matching duo had a big problem with my husband and me, because we were messy and un-ironed looking. We looked like a homeless couple with kids.

How did I get here, really? I grew up watching my mother dress nicely and iron everything. My dad wore suits and knew how to dress with class. My sisters and brother dress sharply. What in the world happened to me? Was I trying to keep street-people looks alive? I made a promise to myself today that I would in the course of six months turn my life around. One day I plan to visit that church looking so respectable that people will wonder if they met me before. You know what? I won't be wearing a dirty shirt that is too small for me. I want to look great like those women who sell clothes in ads that come in the mail.

Sometimes in my need to get my children ready, I completely forget about me. Yesterday I got the kids dressed, fed, and off to school. I went to the store after dropping them off. It occurred to me that I went grocery shopping and forgot to brush my hair or teeth. Fear swept over me like a cloud. I wondered how I could forget to put socks on in thirty-degree weather. Was I losing my mind or just missing a few moments of me time? The answer was clear. I need more time to beautify me. Brushing my hair was not a choice but a necessity. I do chores about 95% of the time. I am always picking up messes, leaving no time to socialize or just laugh. I wish I could let go for a while. I wish I could allow myself to have fun instead of always wanting things to look clean and perfect. It seems that I am compulsive and need order all the time. I am actually jealous of those who can let those dishes sit and then go have fun with the kids.

I listened to a song yesterday as I drove down the road. I sang it loudly from my car. I wondered if I too had turned into a cold parent who was too busy to take time for my kids. I wish I knew how to enjoy life.

Do you know what I think about myself? I see someone invisible to the outside world. No one would notice me if I were gone. How in the world could I have become so unimportant? I guess you have to be someone great to matter much. I think I have always been the invisible person in society to whom no one cares to talk or know more than an hour of his or her life.

I walk around people at the store and they never notice that I am there. I can stand and watch and listen to conversations, and people still never make eye contact with me. How could people be so involved in themselves that they can't see a human standing around them? What does it take to change my life?

If I started wearing bright colors, would people notice that I am lonely and need to talk or need a friend? What if I laugh loudly for no reason? Would someone want to speak to me, or would people think I was a loony person and need to run away from me? The real pain in my heart is that no matter whom I speak to, people don't feel the need to know me one more moment. I wonder if the next person I am kind to will be my new friend. It doesn't work that way. Unless you work with someone, people just don't blurt out, "Hey, let's be friends." After school years and college experiences are over, friendships become difficult to attain.

It has been emptiness without anyone around me. If I were magical, I would create some perfect friends to hang out with who would like me unconditionally and call me daily.

The reality is that life is different for everyone. Loneliness can exist in people my age, not just the elderly. I truly am lonely in my life. Everyone I know is too busy to talk to me on the phone or they don't like me enough to speak to me in person often. I am like the type of food that that you don't want to have too much of, or you will get ill. People limit how much time they spend with me or talk to me. I think it's because I ask too many questions or I am too nosey. It is not that I am trying to be overly inquisitive. I am convinced that like both my children, I have autism. I believe I have Asperger's Syndrome.

I can't get off a subject or questioning, even if I try. I get stuck there like a broken record. Next thing I know, whoever I was hanging around no longer likes me, because of my lawyer style of questioning. I wish I could tell people that I am truly unable to stop this form of communication, but they don't stick around long enough for me to explain. I suffer from severe depression, as well as this communication problem. It has left me without friends, and I don't know if I can ever truly make them and keep them. My children struggle with social and communication problems all the time. They are children, so they don't know I have the same problems.

My whole life I hid things from people. My teacher told me I was dyslexic; I never told my parents. The school put me in reading classes and said I was slow, but they later realized that my reading disability was temporary. I was very determined and learned things the first time I heard them. I learned by fully listening to the teacher, not reading the textbooks. My dependency on hearing what I learned was a weakness. Not often did the teacher have time to cover all material verbally. As I grew up to be an adult learner, I still had problems reading. I tried hard to understand everything well. It always bothered me when people called me smart. I knew I wasn't at all, because it took so much effort to learn the material. Just hard working student I was, nothing more.

The Ashamed

When you're fat like I am, sometimes those we love are just plain ashamed to be seen with us. I was talking with my son the other day, and he says, "Mommy, please do not go to one more Tiger Cub meeting." I quickly wanted to know why, and he said, "Because of how fat you are." I wasn't sure what to feel, anger or sadness. I did look hideously fat. My son, at forty pounds, saw me as an embarrassment. My son had said it many times before. Once he said to me that he did not want me to substitute teach at his school, because his friends made fun of my raincoat and fat.

When I look in the mirror some days, I see someone great. I felt as if I were someone supportive and willing never to think of myself, in order to make people happy. I kept asking myself, "Where did I go wrong with my son?" I felt my son seemed to be ungrateful for all the parties I had attended at his school, all the e-mails I sent to his teacher making sure he was treated fairly. I am one of those mothers who will fight for the rights of my children everywhere. I believe in them, and I believe in protecting them. I wish I could do the same for myself.

I think my heart is broken because I want to be perfect and someone my son is proud of. I didn't raise him to judge or dislike those who are obese. Somehow it existed in his mind that fat is bad.

As I sat in my pool of self-pity tears, I remembered last year, when my son asked me not to wear the raincoat when picking him up at aftercare. He said the kids were making fun of him because of me. This situation made me feel sad for him.

I remember one specific time in my mother's sewing career when she had to iron clothes of a woman whose waist was sixty inches around. Yes, five feet around, and she was five feet tall. Little did I know I would end up just as large as she was. Not once in my life did I make fun of another human being for any reason. Why does it feel I am paying for something, being fat?

Today was the day that I feel that I can't deal with another insult about my weight from anyone. Tomorrow, the thirteenth of January, I will go on a drastic change for the better. I will go to the store and buy diet pills or water pills. I feel like a city water tower at the moment and feel that it would benefit me to buy water pills. Tomorrow. I know that sounds like what all dieters say, but I mean it, diary. I mean it this time.

I have a plan that includes drinking shakes the way I have seen celebrities do. I have plans of being the beautiful wife with perfect clothes and hair. I want to be the feminine woman that I know I can be. It is time to find myself again. She is inside of all this fat. I weighed in at 228 today, and it seems that my weight continues to haunt me every week. Help me, Lord, to fight whatever enemy it is that is taking over my mind and body. I find I hate myself more than a person should, these days.

I looked in the mirror at my side view. All I can see is rolls of fat. I can't tell where my stomach ends and my gut begins, and it all looks confusing. I am very far from looking perfect and celebrity beautiful. I wonder what it must be like to be skinny and wonderful in the eyes of a camera. I have a dream of going to Hawaii and wearing the perfect bathing suit that doesn't scare people with fat rolls.

I have a dream of being skinny in a family photo, where I am not trying to suck in my face while smiling. I have always been jealous of those pretty moms who look great in Easter clothes and always seem perfect, even when cooking. I want that for myself, to be the perfectly happy skinny wife and mom. For now I am a frumpy, unhappy wife.

I want to be the person that I dream of. She has friends that like her for all different reasons. I had a friend who seemed not to like me because he saw I was fat from a photo. We were great friends until he found out I wasn't skinny or hot. That hurt me more than I can tell you. So what if my heart is good and I can keep a great secret? That didn't matter to him. All he saw was someone who didn't work out and someone who got older. He wasn't alone in that shallow world of thinking. Everyone I tried to be friends with held weight standards as a friendship wall.

If someone needs a full body photo, they judge.

The Dress

My husband and I came up with the same idea, to buy two dresses—one dress that fits me and one that is my goal size. Today I did that. I bought a size 0/2 plain velvet dress. Yes, I know it's risky to invest money on clothes I can't wear. The second dress is too little for me as well but the largest size I could find was a twenty at that store, so I quickly called my husband to tell him my plan. He said to me, "You might look like a stuffed sausage in that dress sized twenty right now." When I got home, I quickly put on the dress, and sure enough, he was correct. I looked like a stuffed sausage. I could hardly breathe in it.

I could hear some ripping sounds as I squeezed my huge size twenty-eight self into the size twenty dress. I think it is funny how velvet material feels on the body. I instantly felt like a beautiful princess. I looked in the mirror to think only of the fat green princess cartoon character in a movie, except she turned fat nightly. Yes, I felt like a chunky princess ogre in the dress.

While I was paying for my purchases at the store, the lady behind the counter looked at me and said, "This 0/2 doesn't look anything like what you would fit into." I just smiled and told her that I was going to lose 120 pounds. She smiled at me and said, "You don't need to be this huge; it's bad for your health. I think you can do this weight-loss thing if you try hard enough."

She is right, I can do this. I will lose this weight. Now that I have the pressure of my new dress in the closet, there is nothing in my way. As I sit here typing away, I am sitting in my sausage-squeezed dress feeling pretty. I feel so pretty and like I need new shoes and a purse to go with it.

My daughter is six, and she asks me last night if she and I could wear matching clothes at Easter time. I told her I would think about it. I really want to wear clothes that match my little angel. She is such a special soul and special child to me. I haven't worn a dress since 2000, when I got married. I felt that no one should see me in a skirt or dress because of my huge calves. Once a guy at church made fun of my ankles and calves. You would think that because he was at church, he would have held back on the rude comments, but it didn't protect me that day. He said I had *cankles*, a mixture of fat legs and ankles that looks yucky to most non-chubby-chasing men.

It seems I am setting my goals pretty high these days. I need to lose weight to live longer, but I want to feel accepted and loved too. I have to do this thing now. Guess whom I saw on the television this morning—that guy who lost two hundred pounds running to a restaurant. I don't have that kind of money to go to a restaurant daily, but it sure was cool he represents that company, now that he is thin.

For my wedding I couldn't find a dress. I went to the popular wedding store where women hope to find something cheap. Well, I went there with high hopes. They have beautiful gowns. If I had been small, I would have felt like I became royalty in those dresses. I didn't fit into them. I couldn't find a dress that I could wear that would go over my big super-sized butt. Yes, I said it super sized. Who would ever guess I would be like one of those meals at a restaurant? For my wedding I finally bought a pink dress from a cheap discount store. It wasn't wedding like. It didn't make me feel like a princess. I even made my own veil. I sure hated the way I looked, all fat and chunky on my wedding day. I think every woman dreams of looking beautiful for her wedding day. I just didn't come close to being the person I wanted to be that day. Sometimes I wonder why I allowed myself to get so fat. Who am I hiding from?

Time has slipped by me, and I allowed fat to control everything in my world. I never look at my wedding photos. It bothers me that I didn't have a pretty dress and I didn't feel good about my body. We all deserve to have good moments. I can't say that I have had that many, and it all takes me back to my fat. I hate you, fat self. Leave me alone today. Let me dream of being the perfect person with nice clothes and nice hair and friends. I wish I had friends, but I don't. I have no one to talk to today.

The Photo

I have decided to say something about my photo I accidentally came across today. I think it's hideous, just a photo of me sitting still in a seat. I am not smiling, and I take up a large portion of the four-by-six photo. I look ugly and unhappy. I remember this photo. I had my husband take it a year ago to motivate me to lose weight. Honestly, just between you and me, I'm pretty sure I gained twenty pounds after the photo was taken. I got on the scale today weighing in at 225. Who in her right mind weighs that, being my height?

Diary, you're always there for me. Tell me, where do I go from here? I need to be honest here. The photo was taken by Chris because he was so sick of seeing me frumpy, fat, and miserable. He said that he wanted me to see what he has to look at all the time. It wasn't a compliment, either.

It seems that no matter what's in my diet plan, things go south. When I say go south I don't mean for winter, either. That is a phrase you need to get used to, because, friend, it's my favorite. Going South means my idea is shot and useless. It means that no matter what I tried, it crashed and burned, leaving me at the beginning of nowhere again.

What can I say about that photo that I have not already? I am in an ugly shirt that seems to be the only one I own. Today when I was day-dreaming, I had a funny thought. It was me posing in pictures with all my old clothes. I see that often in celebrity magazines, someone wearing large pants, and you can see the person is half that size. There was only one funny thing added to my daydream that most don't see in a photo. I was flying like superman. I was Super Girl, weight-loss hero. I had a giant *W* on the back of my costume. Can you believe that? When I daydream, I can always be super great and skinny.

Lately while driving, I see a tiny four-inch skinny me doing dances to 1970s music on my dashboard. It is my imagination taking me to weight-loss fantasy world. Am I the only person who sees this skinny version of me dancing in my windshield as I drive? She is laughing at me while I am driving and eating fries from a fast-food place. Did my conscience come out and decide to stare at me from outside my brain? Was I so rude not to listen to her advice that she is now dancing to motivate me? All this time alone is making me see things, and I really need to talk to someone normal right now.

I wish I could talk to someone about what bothers me. I am trapped inside this big giant body, and eating too much is making things worse. I sure want a bag of candy bars right now. They never let me down. Sometimes I think I get high from chocolate and sugar. The feeling I get from eating it makes me feel like nothing could bother me. Candy bar after candy bar, I feel better and better. I have eaten an entire bag of candy while watching TV. It always upsets Chris when I do that.

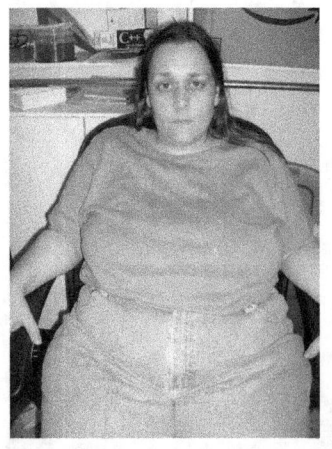

The photo that badly bothered me.

Sometimes I tell my husband he made me fat, and he looks at me and says, "I married you fat." I always say, "No, I was a skinny supermodel when we met." He always laughs and knows to overlook me. I sit here concentrating on the photo. My chest seems to be 48DDD. People get surgery to be large up top. Why in the world is that? My poor back wants me to have

A cups, so I can be one of those athletic-bra-wearing happy runners I saw in Washington, D.C. I remember it clearly as I took photos at the Capital. I counted many neon bras running by me while I took pictures of our great Capital. I thought, "Man, I wish I was flat-chested!" Do those runners have any idea the freedom they get from not being heavy up top? It is probably a blessing to be able to take off running without knocking yourself out. I know what you're thinking; I am too blunt.

Sorry, Diary friend, for my out-of-control sharing. Let me end my comments of the photo I found. It's depressing and looks like I don't own makeup or clothes that I can wear outside of a barnyard. Help me! Can you, please? I bet you could dress me nicely and help me find a way to work out and lose weight. I need a talk-show host to turn me into someone fabulous.

I love daytime talk shows, and I watch them all the time. Recently I have not had the television on much. I am too busy with house chores and the kids to turn on the television. I read all the time how much talk show hosts change lives for the better. I wish I could be useful to the world like that. I'm not sure I could do a talk show, but hey, maybe if I could be a columnist in a newspaper, I would be great at it. I think I am so opinionated that I would be a super great columnist. I like the thought of helping others. I wish I had some great opportunity come along that allowed me to speak to others all the time about depression or problems. Although I can't build myself up at the moment, I feel as if I have the ability to hold others up and help them.

Awards Day

Today was Awards Day at school for the kids. I was very excited to wait and see what both children would get. While waiting I found myself bored and staring at everyone. There seemed to be two kinds of women waiting in the cafeteria: ugly frumpy types, including me, and pretty, sexy mommies. Man, I wish I were like those women who pop out kid after kid only to find themselves in a tiny size-two pants after delivery. I actually had a friend once who did just that.

To get back to what I was telling you, I sat there sick to my stomach watching all those hot mommies hanging out together. They seemed to be ignoring anyone ugly or overweight. They all looked the same, with nice hair, makeup, and clothes. All seemed to dress the same, with tight pants, and the babies seemed to be ignored while the mothers talked up the morning with friends and had happy moments. How rude that seems to me. I tried once to speak to one of those moms at a class party. She sure was snobby to me. I found it to be a waste of my time, fitting in with pretty people. If we were all pulled into a reverse universe one day and everyone was opposite, only then would those who ignore the lonely like me see how it feels.

For years now I have wondered what it must be like to be happy and have friends. There is definitely something different about popular people. They smile more and go out more. They have busy schedules that take them on trips with friends. I watch my sister go on trips all the time, and she sure is popular.

I remember when I was growing up my mother rarely left the house, but then she seemed always miserable. I wonder if she had gone out with friends sometimes, if she would have been happy.

My mother suffered lots of depression, and I think that maybe she too felt like me, lonely for close friends. I don't know; I may be wrong about it. I guess only she could answer that question.

During the awards, I pretended to know the old lady who was sitting beside me, so I started making light conversation with her. She calmly moved herself in the other direction, her back to me. That was not subtle at all, old lady in the expensive coat! I just wanted someone to notice me. Time goes too slowly when you're sitting all alone in some cold cafeteria. I could smell food that I would call mystery meat. I wasn't sure what I was smelling, which is normal for cafeteria food.

We were all sitting on benches made for young children. I heard something crack under me. I think my giant butt broke the lunchroom bench. I hoped I wouldn't land on the floor. I *wanted all the attention to be on my son and daughter, not me. Please God, don't let me cause a scene by breaking this bench by sitting on it.* Thank goodness I wore my blue raincoat. At least I could hide my fears there.

All around me I listened to conversations. I could hear emotions good and bad when people spoke. It's like I can sense if people are angry or sad or happy, even if the words they speak don't match up. Intuition is strong in me these days, but I don't know how to use it. Since I am not part of conversations, I have learned to read people quite well by just looking at them. I am truly bored with myself and life.

One quality that has grown stronger in me is knowing what a person is saying when he or she doesn't respond to a question. I have learned the art of communication through body language and response with all my free time. I watch conversations and can tell when a person is lying by the facial expressions, sometimes, or just the way they speak. Tones of a person say everything, even if the words seem opposite. My loneliness here on earth has given me strengths to understand human behavior and interaction, but I don't know how that skill is useful to me right now.

Now that I seem to have intuition and weird abilities to understand the human mind, I wonder if I will use this later in a workplace or in a relationship. When listening to a person speak, I hear if they like me or not. I can tell if they have sincerity or not. When I noticed someone lying, I have learned to pretend I don't notice. I might freak someone out if I call him or her on all the lies. I will keep all these things to myself for now.

The Books

It was Wednesday. I felt as if the middle of the week needed some extra energy. It seems like days are slower than usual sometimes. I decided to go through the book section of the Walmart store. I am thirty-eight, and I know I shouldn't have been looking in the children's section for books, but my heart was smiling as I read the pop-up Valentine books. I wanted to find the perfect books for my two children. I always like to surprise them on Valentine's Day with a book. Let's face it; there is nothing more pleasing to a six-year old than a pop-up book. Time started to pass as I laughed my way through all the books in the children's section.

While growing up, I loved the bookmobile that would come around to my school. What a wonderful thing it was to be able to see new books to read! If I had been a rich kid, I would have asked for many books, but I honestly knew better than to do that.

To get back to my story, I wandered through the books arriving at ages ten to twelve books. There it was staring at me, science fiction. I could almost hear a voice stating the name of the book. I could hear it calling, "Hey, buy me and read me." I had to move on, because honestly I was not going to buy it. Finally I ended up in the great adult section. No, I don't mean porn books, but I mean cookbooks and the how-to-stay-skinny-forever section of the book area. I couldn't narrow it down to what I wanted to buy today. Was it going to be a vegetarian beginner book or that cool book with secrets? I almost felt pulled to buy that book just to see what was inside it. There I was, not willing to buy anything. I guess I should have gone to the library instead. At least there you can borrow books for a couple weeks and return them. If I were a rich person, I would definitely have one of those official library rooms in my house.

Wait, I can't have a book collection at home, because I am allergic to dust and old things like books. My allergies would keep me from going into my book collection room. My father-in-law loves books and has a room just for his books. He has no idea how bad I feel when I walk into the room of old books. My allergies give me a very difficult time.

I really enjoy reading everything, including newspapers and magazines. In college I said the wrong thing to my professor. He asked what we all loved to read, and I said gossip magazines. Now thinking back, I know that was not the best choice of words for me to use. I should have said I liked scholarly journals, but no, I had to mention my smut magazines by name. Yes, I do love a great magazine with celebrity pictures in it. I like to look at the photos and pretend that I could be that glamorous.

As I was leaving the store without one tiny hint of a book, I thought that maybe the perfect reading material would pass my way soon, but not today. For now I will just search online stores for books on sale in whatever subject I want to read about. My interests this week just happen to be about Egypt and the pyramids. I have a growing desire to visit Italy, too. I think language books might be my interest now.

Something New

Dear Raincoat Diary: I found a coat on the shelf today. it was glowing and magnificent. I had no idea that pretty women's coats existed, since my dear husband bought the only one I ever owned in the men's section of the store. Let me see, my coat is blue and ugly with long arms and well, just yucky. The new coat I found on a hanger was beautiful.

I walked toward the white raincoat, and it spoke out to me. It said, "Buy me, please, before you settle for what you have on again. You deserve to wear me, because I am so nice." I touched the raincoat and thought, *Wow! You are different from the crap I have grown accustomed to wearing around people. What if I wore something so pretty? Would the teacher like me for no reason but my pretty coat? If my daughter were around, would she beg me to buy that and get her a matching one too, along with purses and shoes?* My daughter is everything I wish I could be: classy, and she loves to dress great.

They say the apple doesn't fall far from the tree, and sometimes that is believable, until you're around my daughter. She always sits properly and says polite things. She reminds me of someone who grew up in the right part of society. Her examples must be from shows she watches, since I am pretty sure it wasn't me.

Raincoat, I wish you could always be around, but sometimes I think that people just don't want to see you on me in twenty-degree weather. Today I felt that the bag boy at the store was laughing at me. I did look silly wearing a raincoat on a cold winter day. Sometimes when your pocket holes lose my keys, receipts, and money, I get really angry with you. It's not your fault I don't know how to sew or repair you. You have really been a friend to me, raincoat.

I didn't buy that white beautiful coat today that I saw hanging up. I just kept going. I knew I had only seventy dollars for groceries to last two weeks. It isn't much, when you think about it. The medicine that I take is almost gone, and I don't have money to refill it. I will keep my mouth shut and not tell my husband that I need medicine. He would just get worried about me. He doesn't need to worry about anything more than what he worries about now. We are in debt so far that I don't see us getting out for a while.

My ugly raincoat will have to do for another winter, spring, and summer. That is okay for now, because I don't have friends who visit and I don't have anywhere to go. Are my four walls of my home going to judge me for looking hideous? No, I doubt it. And besides, God still loves me, even if I seem frumpy seven days a week. That is what I tell myself to get through.

As I drove home from my trip to Walmart, I found myself dreaming of the new person that I wanted to be. I wanted to be skinny, nicely dressed, and always classy, just like those movie stars in magazines. My son says that he doesn't want me around his classroom, because the kids laugh at him because I am fat. One day I hope to arrive at a party and have him actually smile and be glad I am around to see him. It's not his fault that I have lost myself in raincoat world and obesity.

Janice

When I was a teenager, I knew a woman in her forties. Her name was Janice. She was overweight and had thick hair and dark eyes. She seemed to be so unhappy with herself that I knew she must have once been a thin person. Sometimes when people are thin their whole life and all of a sudden gain weight, it can be devastating to their spirit. I was only seventeen, and she didn't speak to me very often, because she was my friend's mother. At my young age, I could see life had worn her down. She had six grown children and a couple of grandkids.

Sometimes when I watched Janice cook I could tell that she wished she were doing something more exciting. She had a way about her with her body language that said, "I am miserable with who I am now." She read romance novels for fun and escape. I often wondered why someone would spend so much time indoors reading. For some good reason, she did read book after book. She escaped through cartoon watching too.

Janice must have been American Indian, because she had very dark skin and was from the area of the Carolinas that many would say had Cherokee heritage. I may be wrong, since I never asked her. I often wondered why she seemed to be so shy and unhappy with herself. Now as a thirty-eight-year-old, more than twenty-one years later, I see myself doing all the same things. Life does tire the spirit, especially if chores are all that is left to experience daily.

The woman I knew twenty-one years ago, Janice, didn't like me much. I was quiet and didn't speak to her much. I actually admired her for her hard work and commitment to family. I think I am that way, always putting others first instead of myself, and then I ended up with that tired housewife look on my face too. I wonder sometimes if she lost weight or stayed the same person. I guess we all change throughout the years. I don't live in the same state anymore, so I don't even know if she is still alive.

We never know how we change lives with our behavior. For me she was an example of American married women with children. I think for most wives, life takes its toll on happiness.

Getting off the subject of Janice makes me think of my time at the mill. Now that I think about it, I was wearing a raincoat to work then too. A lady there was in her seventies, and she told me to go to college so I could have a chance at being happy. She said working at the mills was not her plan, but she had no way to leave, with the bills she paid weekly. Well, here I am a college graduate with no clue of how to find my way back to smiling or feeling joys of life.

I have read that being thin makes for a happier person. I know from a lifetime of being overweight that it must be true. I have met some really happy souls, and they all seem to be thin. I don't feel being fat makes me bad, but it adds to my daily worries of health and image in the working world. The world does definitely not unconditionally love me, with my lack of health and clothing style. I feel I make people disgusted with the big jeans and men's T-shirts I wear daily. I fool no one; everyone can still see I am fat.

Reality Check

You know you're fat—I mean really fat—when a couple things occur while in a public place. Here is the best example I can think of. I was at the movie theater with my husband. My husband said he measured me, and I was sixty inches around at nine months pregnant. Now we can't blame it all on baby weight, because the tiny angel was only six pounds. Precious little one, my son he reminded me of a tiny chick, so dependent on me. Anyway, let me get back to my story. My husband decided that I needed to be cheered up by a movie, so we went. I was walking up the aisle to find my seat in the back when all of a sudden I got stuck.

The boys in the theater cleaning—I guess you call them ushers—were pushing the trash can up to clean, and I got crushed between the trash can and the wall. I couldn't believe it. I then tried to sit down, only to find my rear end was way too big for the tiny seats. It was embarrassing. I squished myself into the seat and tried to keep from crying over what had happened to me. I didn't have room to put my arms in the seat with me.

I had the same horrible experience on a plane once on my way to Orlando. I was so heavy that my hips spilled over into the next seat.

It always feels bad when skinny people or healthy people give me that stare. I wonder if it would matter if they knew I don't eat all the time. Sometimes I gain weight without overeating. No one would believe me, I know.

This morning my husband looks at me and says with his hands up in the air about three feet apart that I need to diet. He says that if I ever plan to ride on a plane and not pay for two seats, I better lose weight.

Lately my husband has been quite cruel with his well-meant intentions of helping me. Sometimes I am not in the mood to be reminded that I fail at everything I start. Often I will tell my husband that I am going on a vegan diet. Two hours later, I am tired of it and start eating again.

You know you're fat when your child asks this simple question: "Why do you always wear a raincoat to my classroom?" I always tell him that it makes me happy. He says to me, "Wouldn't it be easier to lose weight than cover it up all the time?" Coming from my seven-year-old, that is an intelligent comment. He got me thinking about my failed attempts at the macrobiotic diet.

I actually read once that many actresses are on that diet, so I figured it was a perfect idea for me. My husband will tell you that my diets last two hours, sometimes four hours, but no longer. I start feeling sick and then I am back to sugar rushes of eating. I honestly think that I eat because it is an addiction. Food doesn't make me feel crappy or let down with harsh words. Food comforts me and makes me feel safe at times. When I have chocolate, I mostly feel happy.

Some have an addiction to drugs, alcohol, or tobacco, but not me. I am addicted to eating food. I always feel a sense of shame afterwards for eating when I really don't need to. I feel jealous of those women who make a decision to look their best and stay on a diet that works. Dear Diary, I am 225 today, and now, twenty-two days into January, I need a friend. I wish I had a friend to talk to.

I know a lot of people and I watch them as they go on trips and go out to eat and to parties. They seem to feel better about life than I do, even if they are chunky too. For more than a decade now, I have searched for a friend, someone I could trust, but friends seem to take from me and then leave out of my life. I am so used to relying on myself that honestly I stopped caring about searching for a best friend to share laughs with. If you're lucky enough to have a friend you trust, hold on to him or her for dear life. It seems impossible to make new friends at thirty-eight years old.It is difficult to meet new people when all I do is shop for groceries. Personally I don't like talking to people while shopping, because my ice cream always melts or I fear my milk is going bad if they ramble on for hours. I think I need a dog to love. They are always loyal and loving. I would pick a black Labrador retriever. I like those dogs so much. I find myself wanting to walk a pet daily. I would love to have two dogs, both Labrador retrievers. I dream of having that, one day. I know that I could love my pets and be great training them. Maybe they would love me and want to be my best buddies. I want puppies that I raise to full-grown dogs. I want them always to have good memories with the kids and me.

The Scary Day

How do I begin to tell you the story of my day? It was a beautiful Saturday. I wanted to take the kids for a few hours outside to play, since they were going crazy being indoors. We love the outside so much. My husband decided that he had plans of his own. He rushed to put his coat on and went outside fast. I could hear him yelling that he was going to burn the Christmas tree. Fear went through my mind, because sometimes he is a little nutty when it comes to starting fires for any reason.

I decided to watch him from the window. He had no luck starting even a small flame on the two-month-old dried tree. I watched him walk to the shed to get something. When he came out I saw a huge container. I wasn't sure if it was gasoline or kerosene. All I knew was it looked like it might be a bad idea. When he put the bucket down, I tried to open the window in the bathroom. I wanted to scream at him not to use that liquid to start the fire. The window was jammed shut. I had never opened it before. What a bad safety issue that was. Anyway, I hit the window hard, but he never heard me.

I watched as he poured two large amounts of the fuel on the small tree. He fired up his lighter and kind of smiled as he saw a flame. Within seconds the flame was like a small explosion. The flame was eight feet high and spread across the yard. It started burning up the yard. I was horrified to see it. I ran to tell the kids that Daddy started a fire and I would be outside for a while helping him. My husband ran into the house and filled some containers with water and went back outside. I ran with him to see if I could help. I asked him if I should call 911, and I thought he said no. I ran back inside to get water to put on the raging yard fire. Why I thought one water pitcher would be enough, I will never understand.

I stomped out the fire with my feet. I could feel the fire on my pants, and I was hoping it would not flame up and burn me too. I had a large rubber container about two feet wide that I was stomping the fire with. I screamed at Chris that I needed to call 911, and he said no again. I did not realize he was saying "Go ahead" instead of "No." I think that when there is a stressful situation, the thought process is not clearly there. I ran in and called 911, and it seemed like it was going to be too late. I ran back outside hating myself for not calling sooner. Why did I think Chris and I could ever put out the fire alone? People in California see this all the time and probably know better than to try to put out a brush fire alone. I was so naïve. Every second that went by, the fire continued to spread and tears were going down my face as I saw my scared kids watch from the window.

It was five feet from our house and closer in the front, and no sign of a fire truck. I was praying for a miracle, because the wind was blowing hard, which fuels a fire. I felt a sickness inside and my asthma was so bad I was hardly breathing anymore. A truck drove by us watching. It was a green truck. I knew who was in it. He never got out to help us; he just sat in his truck watching us run around afraid. My favorite birds, the crows, sat lined up watching the whole thing. They looked sad for some reason. I have always been spiritually connected to nature and birds. I love them around me.

Some volunteer firemen came eventually, and stood at the road watching the fire. I was still struggling to put out the fire going toward the back yard, and my husband was using a water hose to protect the front of the house. By then the entire front yard was burnt completely. We both saw trees flame up instantly and felt the sadness of it all. The firemen got in their trucks and left, never once trying to help put out the fire on the side of the house. Let me tell you, it is difficult to put out a fire without a hose or anything other than a plastic tub. I finally got the fire out on the side, and just in time, because it was headed for my shed. "God save me and the kids." I kept saying this prayer in my mind. I knew that if the house burnt, we had no money to stay in a hotel or any savings to move somewhere new. Like most Americans, we live paycheck to paycheck, barely getting by, because of credit-card debt and everything else.

When we finally got the fire out, my husband and I could not look at each other. We were both pretty angry about what happened. It was stupid for my husband to light fire to a Christmas tree. I am pretty sure he was angry at himself for doing it and putting fuel on it. He asked me not to tell anyone about it, so Raincoat Diary, I am telling you, because it's bothering me. Half an acre burned black that day. Every time I pull into my drive I see it and am reminded that it was a big mistake my husband made. Sometimes I think the common sense part of his brain is missing.

I wish the grass would mysteriously grow back so I could stop seeing that day over and over in my mind. Thank goodness it didn't spread to the adjoining lots behind and beside our house. It burnt only our yard. What have I learned from that scary day? That I don't want to have a real Christmas tree in my house ever again, after seeing how fast they burn. It will be an artificial one from now on. I can now see a pretty yard in back and black yard in front from my window. It's like two separate worlds, light and darkness. I wait, hoping that the next rain will wash away the black ashes of yard that sit there bothering me.

The birds seem to be a bit disgusted with the yard and won't land on it. I don't blame them. They probably don't want black lung disease.

While putting out the fire, not once did I focus on how ugly I was or how fat I was. I was doing whatever it took to protect my family and home. I learned a lot about myself that day, that I am stronger than I thought I was. I will fight to the end to protect those I love. I am Raincoat Super Hero Lorrena. Am I taking it too far?

Super Bowl Day

I went out in my raincoat today. It was Super Bowl Sunday. The stores were so crowded that I didn't even make the effort to get out of the car and try to buy bread at the store. The sun was shining, which made me feel much better than when I first woke up. I haven't fully awakened from this morning. I guess it is because I have been sick for a week.

Today is the first day of February. I don't even want to get into the fact that I failed terribly at starting my diet in January. The pressure to study for my Praxis II exam in March has taken over my life. I study intently at night while the children are asleep. I am so tired. I have no idea if there is even a chance that I will pass. I think that I would be a wonderful social studies or government teacher. It is funny, really, to think that I may very well end up becoming a teacher after all this time. I am so tired from studying facts and timelines.

I am looking forward to the Super Bowl because it is supposed to have some 3-D commercials, and I made sure to get those cool glasses at the grocery store just for the commercials. I know what you're probably thinking, that this is terribly lame. Well, it is, but I want Super Bowl Sunday to be exciting. I got football-shaped Little Debbie brownies for the kids, and I am happy about that. I bet it will be hard to sell football-themed things after the Super Bowl is over. Tomorrow is Groundhog Day, and I am going to guess Mr. Groundhog will see his shadow. I think he will because he often does. Besides, I honestly think we will have winter six more weeks, no matter what the animal sees.

I am like most Americans; I love traditions, so Groundhog Day is a big deal for me, like many other holidays. I think that it will be a couple more times of snow on the ground before it seems like spring is anywhere nearby. Thank goodness I have my raincoat ready to face a new spring. I have twenty-five days until Publishers Clearing House picks a ten-million-dollar winner. I really want it to be me. I could then go to a dentist and take the kids to a dentist.

I have dental insurance, but it covers only eighty percent of the costs, and I never have the other twenty percent to pay the cost of going to the dentist, so we never go. Sad really, to think that insurance doesn't help at all. I wonder how many Americans feel the same way I do. It would be nice to have extra money. I finally did it. I put the kids in aftercare, so I could take teaching jobs at school as a substitute. I feel a bit afraid of change and not being there for the kids daily. I am always the one who is there to pick them up. Waiting and waiting is definitely a pain in the rear. I won't miss sitting in my car freezing in the middle of winter. I will miss seeing their little faces smiling back at me.

Last week I had to turn down at least six jobs, because I had no aftercare for the kids and couldn't take all-day jobs, because of how long they lasted. Now that I have aftercare, I can take a job every day of the week. The only downside of it all is the sheer fact I can't study for the Praxis Exam and have no idea when I will be capable of doing it. I pray for a miracle for passing that exam.

It's always a risk to make changes in one's life. For me I really need job experience. I am hopeful that working at the junior high schools and high school will give me references that I truly need to get hired later on as a licensed teacher. I used to say to people that I would never consider teaching or setting foot in a school building. I guess I shouldn't have been so sure about it. I am eating my own words.

The Substitute

This week I was the lonely substitute. Many of the kids were abusive to me. I think I gained more weight this week than in previous times. I don't show anger or emotions like others. It's like it's trapped inside that cement brain of mine, all waiting to escape, like fumes. What is there to say other than this week was terrible? Many of my students took ten bathroom breaks an hour. Everyone held phones and MP3 players in their hands like it was normal to have them in class. When I was growing up, school meant that I was going to learn something new. Not now, according my experience. The kids show up in class and hope to do nothing. Many ignore the assignments and talk to friends like they are at the mall. I feel like I am invisible at school, being a substitute. I wish I were respected and the kids would listen to me.

I learned something about teens this week. It seems the ones that kiss butt and pretend to be kind to me are the worst-behaved students. Most of the troublemakers volunteer to clean the room and take roll. They know what to do to stay in good with the teachers. As a substitute I found that the good students, the ones who really study and listen, have very few friends. I watched the behavior patterns of those who were dumb, ugly, even downright crazy. Always the same: their behavior was aggressive and they picked on the meek, kind kids. Sometimes

I could even see a glimmer of myself in the meek ones. I wish I were rich. I could then own my own business. I think I would own a singing telegram business or a flower shop.

It is almost time for Valentine's Day, and I wonder how many wonderful roses will be given away. I dream of being one of those lucky women who gets pink roses on Valentine's Day. I never get flowers from anywhere. I would like to get flowers and smile the way people smile when they get them. I saw a show once where a guy delivered flowers to a complete stranger because he saw her crying. It was a perfect idea, doing that.

Substitute teaching is not good pay, and I wonder if it will supply enough money to buy school lunches for the kids or even buy groceries. It's always scary to think about bills. Bills are too high in the wintertime, because of heating.

Today as I tried to teach algebra, some kid was playing his acoustic guitar. He ignored his assignment and pretended he was home alone. That situation made me feel bad, because the students treat me as if I'm invisible.

One kid kept making fun of my weight. He was a football player. He kept saying I was fat, and he could tell I never exercise. Well, Sherlock Holmes, you really figured out something when you saw I was lazy and fat. I wish I could wake up skinny and begin running five miles a day. Yes, I would like to be fit like marathon runners. That would be cool. I would wear only a tank top and shorts on my run. I am kidding about the tank top. I would probably wear the most covering shirt I possibly could. I am very conservative all the time.

I listened as I substituted today. The kids at school spoke of how they would starve, to stay in a certain weight class in wrestling. The cheerleaders would laugh about how they eat only 500 calories a day to stay skinny. I remembered being this way myself as a teen. How did I forget all the important things to staying fit and thin through the years? I wish I could be a tiny bit the way I was as a child. All these kids remind me of just how old I am. They all seem so young and have their lives ahead of them. They just don't know it.

Windy Day

Have you ever just stood with the wind blowing on your face? Today the wind blew softly. It wasn't blowing in a way that would mess up my hair or knock over stuff in my backyard. It was the perfect day, full of warmth and sun. I decided that I would take out the kites for my children and have a great day. Both kites were only a dollar. I took out the kites and wondered how I could get them to fly. Within minutes the wind picked up the kites without any help at all. I couldn't believe how well they took off flying.

I stood and watched the trees blowing and everything felt good to be around. I love nature and birds in my life. I wondered what it must be like to be suffocated within the confines of the city with no space. I was standing on several acres of land, with no one around for a long way. Living in the country sure has its benefits.

I was standing in the yard happy to be able to see the big blue sky above me. Four crows sat in a tree watching as my family and I enjoyed being outside on a Saturday. A few times a bird tried to fly near the kite, and it was funny. The kite kept taking a nose dive into the ground after being up as high as it could go on the string. I had to tell my daughter to watch out for the nose-diving kite, because it looked scary on its way down to the ground.

It is only February, and I feel ready to see flowers and sunny skies again. The winter wasn't harsh, but it was gray. An inspiration came to me while I was out in the wind, and that was to plant a few trees. I think that red- and pink-blooming trees would be wonderful. I made a fast inventory of all that surrounded where I live, and all I could see was green. I think I need colorful plants around me now. Funny thing is that today I don't feel like putting on my ugly raincoat, and it is rare for me not to want to put it on.

I have come to terms about my raincoat. It is like my blanket. I carry it around for security. Who would ever think that a woman in her late thirties would need something like that to feel safe? Well, me, I guess. The best thing about my windy day was that I didn't feel overheated or suffocated. My asthma didn't bother me at all. Today it was an inviting day for me to feel happy for a moment. It was truly the perfect day with my kids and the kites outside in the sun. My soul felt free for once in my life.

Today I didn't need my raincoat, and I didn't care that I was over-weight. I just enjoyed my life and moments with my kids.

Addiction

Sometimes I wonder if anyone knows what his or her addiction is. For some I think it is sex, the Internet, or maybe drugs or alcohol. To me the true definition of an addiction is something that you feel you can't live without. Last year it was friends. I couldn't seem to function unless I felt I had friends. I have heard of many alcoholic-support groups. What about the rest of our addictions? How do we fix them? I mean really, first we must admit we have one.

Raincoat Diary, I am going to be honest for once this week. My addiction is chocolate at the moment. Somehow when I am down and feeling like the whole world is against me, I get a hint of thought that a chocolate bar will make everything better. I even convinced myself there were healing qualities of caffeine and antioxidants every time I ate a candy bar.

It never occurred to me that my spouse saw my addiction as a threat until yesterday. We were watching TV, and I said to him calmly, "Can you go get me chocolate?"

He quickly said, "No way. I am not in the mood to lose you this year."

I felt upset with him, because he quickly brushed off my request. I tried to find ways to get him to go to the store, like making up excuses. I said that we needed milk and bread and toilet paper. I knew if I could get him to go to the store that maybe I was one step closer to getting what I needed for my addiction. He continued to say that I wasn't getting one sweet thing this weekend. I was angry with him.

We were in the car on our way back from the gas station, and I said to him, "Why wouldn't you stop and get me a stupid candy bar? It will make me feel better." I was feeling nervous at that point.

He looked at me quickly by pulling his eyes off the road and said, "You're a fat cow. I don't want a fat cow in my life." He went on to say, "Fat cows die, and you will die this year, if you keep gaining weight."

I was shocked. After all I did for him, cleaning, cooking, and raising the kids, was it all for nothing? All he could see was a FC. I reduced that name to two letters, to feel better.

When we got home, my seven-year-old son tried to make me feel better. He said that I wasn't one fat cow, but my body looked like two skinny cows connected together. My son said all I had to do was lose one skinny cow, and then I would look great. It didn't make much difference. I think something inside of me snapped. My husband was right about me. I am a fat cow and need to lose weight before I die of a heart attack. The truth doesn't make me feel happy at all. My husband was cruel to me. He was not accepting, just like everyone I had tried to be friends with. No one loves me, and I deserve this.

While I was teaching as a substitute, the children would taunt me with comments about being fat.

I made a promise to myself that I would never let my husband hurt me again as bad as he hurt me with that comment. I would shut off that side of my heart from him. The reality is that I have a strong addiction to chocolate.

When he didn't get me the candy bar, I went behind his back and made a very strong chocolate drink with pure cocoa.

As I sit here wondering about my life, all I can think of is that I wish I were skinny and perfect. I wish that I didn't rely on chocolate or the coat to make me stronger. I really am jealous of those who can take their goals anywhere. I want to run like those marathon runners. I want to be skinny and not obese like I am now. I resent my husband for being so cruel. I wish he could understand what it's like to be me.

February

Here we are, the most romantic month of the whole year. Everyone will be getting flowers and candy for Valentine's Day. My husband doesn't think I deserve candy because I am fat. I like to hear about others' romantic getaways to places like the ocean. I'll bet celebrities have the best Valentine's Days ever.

I thought I would write you because I have no one to talk to. If I could plan the perfect Valentine's Day, it would have pink roses that showed up at my door and surprised me. I love pink more than red. I always loved that type of flower in pink. My perfect Valentine's Day would have balloons and a cute bear holding candy. The good candy should be with the bear, not that nasty stuff that tastes like plastic. Good candy is the kind that had a name you recognize.

The perfect Valentine's Day would have a romantic dinner with Italian food. I don't remember the last time I ate Italian food. There would be great music playing during my meal and lots of conversation. There is nothing more romantic then a guy who can carry on a conversation about anything.

Valentine's Day to me is all about love and showing the person you're with how much he or she means to you. I haven't ever felt that holiday was shared correctly with me. It speaks for itself, I guess.

Sometimes when I am at work and a lady gets flowers, I get jealous and wonder what she did to deserve those. I wonder if she will take the flowers home and put them in a vase or throw them out on the way to her car.

I would like to wake up one morning and be loved and have hundreds of friends. Well, maybe a few friends are fine, too. I would invite my friends over to show them my beautiful flowers I got for Valentine's Day. I would share a toast with them and laugh at almost anything. I have another definition for Valentine's Day, and it is passion. Passion exists in everyone, I think, if they are with the right person. If you marry the wrong person, you might not feel it at all. I know many women like that.

In school Valentine's Day means looking at all the cards you got from classmates and seeing who likes you or doesn't. I am at home and will probably not receive cards from anyone. I will probably turn on the television and hope that morning shows have some great Valentine stories for me to watch. I vicariously live through happy couples' lives I see on TV.

Today is Valentine's Day. I wonder how many people will be going somewhere. I got my kids boxes of candy and cards. I also got them giant stuffed bears. I got my husband a large box of candy and a card. I waited eagerly while everyone was giving cards to each other. The kids and I stared at my husband, wondering what he got me for the holiday. The answer was nothing. I asked him where my candy was, and he said he thought I could get myself something, since I have access to the bank account.

Disappointment came over me when I thought how cold my husband was for not even getting me even a stupid card. I should have expected such rudeness, since for the last nine years, there have been no pink roses for me. I love those flowers. I never preferred the red ones, because they don't seem to make me happy.

I quickly went to my e-mail to see if any so-called friends sent me an e-mail card. No one thought enough of me to do it. I imagine that I will think twice about remembering them for any reason on the next holiday. It seems that women put so much thought into stuff, and we always think our man will reciprocate, but he doesn't do anything sometimes. I would like to know why God made men and women so different when it comes to relationships.

Valentine's Day is always one of those holidays men dislike because they have to get flowers and candy and jewelry. I imagine if men could keep one holiday from happening, it would be Valentine's Day. Dear Raincoat, if I could wear you today, I would, but it's sunny and warm. Maybe then I would feel good, but for now I feel sad that I didn't get cards or e-cards from any friends. Mother did surprise me and sent me an e-card, and that gave me a smile.

I have decided I hate Valentine's Day. It's for happy lovers, and that doesn't include me. Next year I think I will not celebrate it with twenty balloons and decorations around the house like I did this year. My son says that I go overboard all the time, and he is probably right. Why should I care anymore, if no one else notices? I cleaned the entire house for Valentine's Day, and no one noticed. I am actually not a depressive, even if it seems that way to outsiders. I am able to feel a sense of happiness today because I am alive and can hear and smell and experience the world around me.

Tomorrow will be much better. I have new secret plans for weight loss. I plan to start my diet and exercise program tomorrow. My current weight could kill me at 228. There is no stopping me. I know I can make this happen, the weight loss. I will promise myself that every person who has hurt me along the way with my weight will not be part of my life anymore after I am skinny, with exceptions to my boy. I will always love him with all my heart.

Maybe everything won't feel so final, and maybe I will forgive all those shallow friends who hate me because I am fat. I do know that some are ignoring me because they like only thin friends. It is those that I will snub once I am skinny and fit. I can do it thanks to a show about weight loss I watch intently every week. I believe that one day I can be successful just like those people. Fat doesn't have me anymore. I can lose it, and I will. I am making a wish for myself this Valentine's Day. I wish to be 128 pounds skinnier and to find new, wonderful friends. I wish to find the perfect job. I want everything I do to be a success. I can do this.

Friday the 13th

Personally I love the number thirteen. It's always been a familiar number to me. When I have to grab a number at the DMV or anywhere else, I always somehow get that number. When I run toward my microwave to turn off my boiling-over burnt food, it stops on thirteen. I have no problem with that number, unlike many people. Don't get me wrong; I am superstitious, but not in the way that most are.

When I see a black cat running away from my path, I always say to myself that it means good luck. Most people would say what kind of curse are you under if black cats run away from you? I think most of the time my husband thinks I am cursed. He says if something weird or unusual is going to happen, it will be when I am around. I choose to believe the opposite. Sometimes I pretend I am very lucky. I like to think that cats are preventing me from having bad luck by running away fast instead of going across my path.

Today is Friday the thirteenth, and I feel fabulous. The air is cool and the birds are singing in the trees around my house. I was walking around listening to sounds when I found a woodpecker in a tree. Then I found two birds of the same species. Both seem to be pecking away at the innocent tree. I wondered if they would kill my poor trees in search of bugs to eat. Today I saw a cardinal and a few robins. My favorite friends the crows came by to say hello. They always watch me from the trees. I saw a hawk flying down near me in one fast swoop. I said to the bird, "Sorry, buddy, I am too big to eat for lunch and carry off to your nest."

The day was going fine, even though my husband asked me not to drive anywhere, because it was the thirteenth of February. I was walking up to my front door when all of a sudden I looked down to see a dead bird beside my door. Thoughts rushed through my head and I wondered if it was some sign. Was the dead bird a sign that something bad was coming? Did the dead bird mean that my neighbors hated me? Why was the tiny little creature dead and stiff lying where I could see him? There wasn't a tree anywhere in sight, and it didn't fall from a nest like a baby bird.

Insecurity struck my mind instantly. What if I killed that innocent bird when I threw out some round cereal to feed the animals? I thought I was doing my part to help the environment. I fed the animals with my uneaten cereal. What if it got stuck in his tiny little beak and he suffocated because of me? Poor dead bird, I wonder how old he was. I took a broom and swept him off my porch thinking that some other animal would carry him off soon. I do have more than my share of dogs walking by during the night.

Speaking of dogs, yesterday while I was watching birds in my backyard, I saw a dog come up and pee in my kids' sandbox. I was very afraid he would poop also in my sandbox. I tried to scare him away, but he peed on the swing set too. I was sad that my backyard had turned into an outhouse for crazy dogs.

I turned on my computer typing fast to find out if there was a bad omen involved with dead birds. All I knew was that it was Friday the thirteenth, and a dead bird was waiting for me at my front door. Another thought crossed my mind. What if the environment killed that bird and he drank some water and dropped dead? Was I the next victim of poor water? Yes, it does seem that the dead bird turned me into Mrs. Paranoid. I did not find much on the Internet about dead birds, other than a list of how it died, such as being attacked by a cat.

I came to a small conclusion about the dead bird today: it just happened to die near my door. There was no meaning behind it, just an animal's time to go.

Memories

When I was growing up, I saw all kinds of people who were overweight. I used to be afraid of them, wondering what terrible thing they did to get that large. I used to be afraid that I would one day be overweight, and here I am obese. I am what I never wanted to be, but I slowly became a fat lady. In social studies class in junior high, I used to think about my teacher's weight. I wondered if teaching social studies made a person fat. Do you know how ironic this all seems, now that I am trying to go into teaching social studies?

What terrible thing did I do to deserve to feel completely miserable like this at 228 pounds? "Help me, someone out there," I wish I could yell and some lady from a weight-loss clinic would show up at my door with a free membership. I am actually wishing I could be one of those early morning runners who never miss a morning of exercise. Despite all the insults that I receive from students I teach and at home, I still lack true commitment to my health and myself.

It is time to be honest about myself completely. I love food more than I love myself. I love the smells and taste of food, especially things with margarine in them. I live every day eating huge amounts of cheese. This habit has indeed contributed to a very fat body. How I want to change and make a real difference in my life! I wish I could learn to love myself as much I love others. I do so much to make my family happy and nothing to try to make myself happy.

Sometimes when I go to church the older ladies stare at my winter coat. It is torn near the pockets and is peeling away in spots. I look like a bag lady on the street in a winter coat that doesn't have a liner. I hate wearing old clothes, and everyone seems to think I am trashy. Every day I think that I can work and earn a couple dollars and buy myself some shoes or a coat, but I don't. I spend the money on things the kids need. I don't have the nerve to buy the things I need.

I look ugly and neglected, mostly with my bad hair that needs to be styled and old torn clothes. I am ashamed to visit people or go to work. When I go to work, I wear shirts that no longer have a hem in them, and I hope that others won't notice. I try to tell myself that materialism is bad and that I will be fine, but the stares from others hurt my soul daily.

Being fat only adds to my lack of fitting in with society. Even in nice clothes, my weight would pour out to everyone, and they would think I was lazy. No one ever asks me if I lost my thyroid. If they asked me, I would say, "Very good observation, because I no longer have a thyroid that works." I want to believe that this year will be the year I lose weight. I have to find a way to change my mental state.

I have compiled a list of things I must do to prepare myself for a new life, so dearest raincoat, I write with secrecy, as I will tell only you this for now. First thing I plan to do is to stop e-mailing shallow friends who I think only use me and never seem to uplift me in any way. I believe that useless e-mail friends only drag me down and make me feel rejected. Today I will put up an emotional wall and not turn around again to emotional e-mail vampires. All are the same; they want me to be their friend, but they never answer my e-mails at all. Good-bye, shallow draining friends. I will not be there for you anymore.

The second part of my new life is to find a time to exercise each day. I thought it would be four in the morning and quickly realized that was not an option, as I am not a morning person. Then I thought maybe I would move my plans to evening, and somehow my chores became too much for me to find time for me. So here is part two of my plan: to get my husband to do some of the chores, so I can have me time. It's not too much to ask that he help.

The third part of my plan is to cut out cheese products and milk products, including butter and ice cream, and one last thing, chocolate. I know I said candy was an addiction to me. I am telling myself over and over out loud that I eat only salads. I eat only salads I'll keep saying it until one day I believe it. Maybe I will wake up feeling like I eat only salads. I think it will take close to one hundred times for me to hear it to believe it.

There is one more part to my plan to lose weight.

I want to play my guitar every day and bring back the part of myself that I so love, songwriting. I love to write songs, and I love to sing. I am finding myself again, and I truly believe I will be the person I need to be by July, my birthday. I will be thirty-nine years old this year, and it is high time I loved who I am, inside and out.

New Day

Here I am, and it is a new day. Current weight 225, and I am ready to take on this fight to save my life. My hips hurt some from being 135 pounds overweight. My goal to reach is a weight of ninety-five. I want to be slim and happy and physically fit. Today is my first day of saying no to things I like. I will say no to cheese and chocolate. Why do things I like start with the letter *C*? I have been saying "No, thank you; I don't eat that" over and over since I woke up at four o'clock. I have been saying quietly to myself, "I eat only salad, chicken, or unsweetened cereal."

I will take control of my body today, and I will win. I am determined not to let my weak side win. If I have a bad day with the kids fighting and being bad, I will not run to the refrigerator and fill my anxiety with food. This is my problem, and I will face it prayerfully. I have begun to understand something really important today. The fat I see on myself, others see too, and it looks terrible. I will think positively from now on to win this battle of obesity. I don't have anyone to support me on this. I will become my best friend.

I am a good friend, and I will become one for myself. I deserve to look good and feel great. Today is the day I will become a new person. I know I said the same thing at the beginning of the year, but somehow today I feel different.

I have a hidden candy bar in the kitchen. I will give to one of the kids so I won't eat it when I feel weak. Candy is a drug to me that I must kick. I can't be living for food anymore. My heart is hurting daily, and I wonder if I will leave my children behind because of a heart attack. I can't allow my health to fail me now.

I can't keep wearing my security raincoat to cover up fat. I have to face the truth about myself, that I am dangerously overweight. I will need prayers and I will need dedication from myself this time. I am wearing jogging pants today. I am going to exercise and burn fat today, even if I don't feel like it. No one can help me except me, when it comes to controlling what goes into my mouth.

My mom used to say when I was growing up all women put their jeans on the same way, but some just look better in them. My mom always dressed and looked healthy. I wish I were more like her. She always ate the right foods, and I wish I had paid more attention to that. She stayed skinny and healthy.

Today is my day to shine. Yes, February 16, 2009, is the first day of my new life.

Some kids in school where I substitute teach have been cruel to me when I go up to the chalkboard to write something. I can hear the snickers and laughter about my body size. I don't blame them, really. I am huge, and it is time I accept that truth about myself. People are cruel. My husband says he is cruel to me because he wants me to lose weight. After hearing insults from everyone I see, it has no meaning to me. It rolls off my mind like it never happened.

I often look at skinny models and actresses and say to myself that they didn't really have to work to get where they are, but maybe I am wrong. Maybe all the actresses out there have personal trainers, and maybe they all try very hard to look fantastic. Putting in the hard work is something that I need to do now for weight loss.

My husband wants to see our families in another state in just under a month. I am afraid to go visit them now at my highest weight. I am afraid that Dad would feel ashamed of me. I am worried my sisters will be sickened by my weight. They will not say anything mean, though.

Weight keeps me from going out in public. I tell myself that I don't need to be at the bowling lanes, because you have to walk up with a ball and roll it. While you're bowling, everyone can see your behind. I am not sure I want that right now, so I make excuses of why I cannot bowl. If we are going to a restaurant, I tell my husband that we should go pick up the food and bring it home instead of going in to eat. I have anxieties that those in restaurant will think I am unworthy of eating anything.

I want to be normal, but I just can't be, right now. I sure wish I had a weight-loss person coaching me and helping me along. I feel alone every day of my life.

Today I think ahead and dream of getting my weight under control and weighing fewer than 200 pounds at first. I always dreamed of being beautiful. It is not anyone's fault that I am fat. I beg my poor husband to buy me candy and give him no choice. I tell him if he loves me, he will go get me the candy.

The weight-loss shows on TV keep me in the mental state that I can do anything. I try not to miss a show. Those people are really lucky to have a personal trainer like that. I would love to be on that show. The only fear of being on it would be when they have to weigh in wearing only athletic bras and stretch pants. My husband says stretch pants and I don't go together well at all. He feels sick when I wear stretch pants in public.

I had my husband put the mirror down lower on the wall last night. Since then I have been sickened by the views I see of myself. I had no idea I looked like that to him and the kids. It was easy to be fat if I didn't see anything but my face in the mirror. He moved the mirror low enough for me to see my whole body. That really made me aware of my problems. A reality check is now my mirror that looks at me every time I leave my bedroom.

I don't think mirrors lie at all, so I have to face the fact that I am ugly right now. I don't have friends, and I don't have people to talk to every day, so here I am writing you, Raincoat Diary. If I did have friends I could talk to daily, I think I would feel better. That is not an option at this point, so I will just deal with it.

Here are the facts: I am obese and I am scared of my favorite foods and I am afraid of my appetite ruining everything. I got some diet pills that don't seem to do much of anything. I looked at all the breakfast cereals, and they are covered in sugar. I looked at Pop Tarts and other stuff in my cabinet and feel too nervous to eat them. I will go back to my original statement to myself. I eat only salads. I should start to believe it soon.

Being Very Sick

I started out my week feeling like I could do anything. I worked day after day at a job I really dislike but kept my spirits up. I told myself that making a living is required, and I should not complain. Then Friday February 20 appeared out of nowhere. I woke up to feeling as if I had no ability to breathe. I had a migraine along with flu symptoms. To beat all this, my six-year-old was ill. I kept her out of school because I was worrying. The entire day she watched over me like an angel.

As I lay still on the couch feeling like a bad mommy, I tried not to move at all. All the sounds of the outside world were tearing at my brain. My headache was here to stay; I could tell. As hours went by, I wondered if I would have the strength to drive and pick up my child from school. I hoped that my husband would take a work day off and help me, but he did not. I found the inner strength to get off the couch and drive to the school. I don't think anyone would have understood how sick I was that day.

The next day was Saturday, and we had four different events we had to take care of. We went to a birthday party that lasted two hours, and the party wasn't even over when we left. We also went to a banquet that evening. I wish I hadn't attended, because I did two very embarrassing things. I coughed water all over everyone while they were eating, and then I fell out of my chair onto the floor. My hip was hurt, but I pretended to be fine. I was so weak I couldn't believe I was spending time at a banquet when I should have been home in bed. I think it took its toll on my body, because the next few days were rough for me.

Day after day I coughed and coughed and tried to find a way to breathe. I made a big mistake by deciding to go to the doctor's clinic. The clinic took more than five hours to see me, and I managed to pick up other illnesses while waiting in the room with other patients. I have come to the conclusion that I am a sponge. I absorb others' illnesses as quickly as possible. Nine days later I am still sick from bronchitis and wondering if I will ever stop coughing and feeling ill. I am almost out of antibiotics and cough syrup, and I feel like I never got better at all. There was one good thing from this illness. I lost about ten pounds of weight because of my bronchitis.

With the new weight loss, I feel better from less-tight pants. I still felt a need to grab my buddy the raincoat today, but I do know that weight loss is the key to a better way of life. If ten pounds can make me feel better, then one hundred can make me feel free and fantastic.

I don't have a coach telling me to eat right or a friend to walk me through the tough times. I have a couple weaknesses right now. One weakness is stress eating when the kids fight or my husband is yelling at the kids. My other weakness is soft drinks. Sometimes I drink one to feel better and the sugar and caffeine make me feel like everything is going to be okay. I find simple pleasure in drinking a beverage.

I forced myself to read articles on foods and what is really in them to discourage myself from putting things in my mouth ever. I am pretty sure I won't touch yogurt again after reading that red bugs were in it. Why does the truth always bother me so much? I was perfectly happy not knowing what secret lurked inside my favorite snacks. I am still kicking myself wondering why I need to be so darned informed about everything. Food shouldn't have secrets at all. Now I feel compelled to research all my favorite foods.

Eating For No Reason

Today I ate five meals by one p.m. How do I explain this behavior, other than stress eating? I eat when I am upset, and this week is tough. My daughter and I both have pneumonia, and this is my third week being ill. I started my day by making meals for my sick daughter. Her weight dropped, and I have been trying to find something she will eat. When she says, "No, I don't want anything," I feel guilty and eat what I prepared.

Now here I sit knowing that when I get on that scale I will have gained two or three pounds today. Yesterday I gained two pounds and felt like a bad person. Today here I am, the same problem over and over. I wish I had a friend to talk to about this problem of mine. Sometimes I wish I had lots of money so I could have a physical trainer in a gym to teach me all that I need to know about fitness. Then I wonder where would be the time for me even to drive over to a gym and work out. Every moment of the day is taken by chores.

Today I did lots of loads of laundry because my daughter kept throwing up and her clothes and blankets were dirty. I found that every minute of the day brought more responsibilities. Being sick myself, I find that I have no energy to laugh or to smile. I feel like sleeping. I have a test to take for teaching in a little more than a week, and I know in my heart I am not ready to take the test that lasts more than three hours. I wish I could be a genius and remember everything I read the first time. I am definitely far from a genius and will struggle to remember even tiny facts for the tests. It will take some sort of test miracle for me to score high enough to pass.

Today I am left with guilt for how much I consumed and how much cheese I found on my plate. I thought my addiction to cheese was over. The first sign of a bad day, and here I am eating cheese on every plate of food, especially spaghetti. I wanted to lose weight and show myself and my family that I am not a loser and fat cow. My kids always joke about my size in public, and sometimes I feel terrible about it. How do I prove to myself that the evil that takes over me—the sin of gluttony—is no longer a challenge to me? I have to overcome this problem of going to the refrigerator whenever I can't handle something.

I watch shows on TV where people have family support, and they just call up a family member and everything is all right. Well, that is not me. I don't live close to family members, and they would be too busy with their lives to hear about my tiny problems. Today more than ever, I need a friend. Where is she right now? I need some friend who needs to lose weight just like me. A skinny person might not understand my dilemma and obsessive behavior.

When I wake tomorrow, I need to look in the mirror and say to myself that I don't need a lot of calories to deal with my day. I already know that I am taking my daughter to the doctor, and that alone is stressful. Waiting rooms full of coughing, sick kids always keep me in a weird mood. I have to drive a long distance for her appointment, so that alone leaves me stressed one day before. Raincoat Diary, I am going to make you this secret promise today before I wake tomorrow. I promise not to eat more than three meals tomorrow, even if I feel angry or sad.

I made a big mistake of wearing stripes today. They always make me feel extra fat. Stripes on a fat lady definitely do not make me feel skinny or pretty. Why did I wear an ugly design today? Tomorrow I will try to wear something a little less ugly. Too bad it is almost spring, and black is not in fashion anymore.

I didn't realize it was possible to gain five pounds in a day, but I managed to do that. I have managed to gain back weight I lost last week starving myself. I guess I shouldn't have stopped eating altogether. When I returned to eating again, the weight came back quickly. I was watching the weight loss show this week and couldn't believe how much many had lost. One guy lost ninety pounds in nine weeks, and I pretended it was me on the show.

I checked my e-mail for days and days, and no friends wrote to me. I know I don't really have friends I see in person, but there are a few e-mail buddies that I sometimes hear from. I am too embarrassed ever to really talk to e-mail buddies about my obesity. It seems that everyone I know is confident and has good relationships with their spouses. I don't think anyone would relate to my life. I kept all this locked in my mind until now. Here I am telling you my deepest secrets.

No one wants to be ugly or fat or unhealthy. I believe that, so why am I trapping myself in this body year after year? I wish I could make it all stop and wake up skinny and fit. I know I am lying to myself when I think fat goes away for no reason.

Goal Night

Guess what, Raincoat Diary. Here I am ready to start over. It is now March 6, for at least a few more hours, and I need change. I need to be less trashy and less ugly. For now I need to search for a brand new job, because substitute teaching is giving me a migraine and an ulcer. I think I need a complete overhaul. Yes, this, friend, is goal night. I will make some life goals that I plan to accomplish.

First I want to meet my favorite artist/singer of all time. That is one of my long-term goals, of course. I quickly went to his website to see where he was touring next. Since I can't travel to other states or countries, I guess I will just have to visit him on my favorite web channel and watch any live videos I can. I love his website too. If I could just meet him, maybe I could stand beside him and sing. Wait! What am I saying? He is talented and probably would not want an extra set of vocals in his wonderful performances. Let me dream for once before you laugh away my idea. I would sing the backup vocals with him for fun on some talk show. He would love me, I hope.

I have to set a goal. I have to be someone great, and I have to change now, or I will melt like a candle from boredom in my life.

The music part of my personality has been suppressed so long I don't even think my husband or kids would know me if I brought that side of me back. It occurred to me one day that I have no hobbies or favorite anything. How on earth can I accomplish happiness if I don't know what happiness is? Well, here I am, ready to set goals for myself.

March 7 happens in only a few hours, and it is my first day being a new person. Will I meet my favorite singer? Well, of course I will. I have to believe that. When I meet him it will be on some television show. Why am I on the show? Who knows? I will worry about that later. For now I am content to have a goal. Now I must find a new way to lose weight, or else I will be frumpy fat when I meet my favorite singer of all time.

Another goal for me would be to have a completely better hairdo. Let's see, do I look good with curly hair or straight? I'm not sure what I need to be right now. I just know it is something new. I am sick of looking like I belong at a homeless shelter and feeling like I have a nasty image everywhere I go. I am jealous of all women who have money to go to a salon and have their hair and nails done. I would love to be pretty and happy like them. I remind myself of some old mill worker that never got out of her situation and always wears a ponytail.

Let me get back to my goals. Tomorrow morning I will refuse to eat. At lunch I will eat only a marshmallow. Wait, maybe I will eat more than that. I am already getting hungry thinking about just one marshmallow as my meal.

I woke up feeling cursed this morning. Every time I grabbed a plate or bowl of food, a hair would be across it to gross me out. The universe sure has tried to keep me from eating. I always just get the eyelash or hair out of my plate and say to myself it didn't happen.

I have a necklace I bought once that is supposed to help me lose weight. All it ever did was jinx my cheese crackers. I opened the bag, and it seemed to be full of pubic hair. I am officially sick to my stomach sharing that story with you, Raincoat Diary. Yes, it is official. I feel like throwing up, and that cheese cracker incident happened more than nine years ago.

Once on a date I saw a dead rat lying on its side near a wall. I was getting ready to eat my chili soup, and all of a sudden there it was, a view of a rat. You would think that I would have gotten sick at that moment, but no. I talked myself into eating my food and blocking it out. I am convinced that I have some evil thing inside my head that keeps me fat. It makes me stronger and more able to cope with disgusting situations. Truly, if Mother had noticed that rat at the restaurant, she would have stopped eating for months. I wish I were more like my precious mom. At least she knows how to stay thin.

Here I am losing track of my goals. My goal for March is to lose twenty pounds. I have twenty-five days to lose that weight. I can and will do this, even if it makes me sick. Tomorrow I will begin by stepping on that horrible scale and facing the music. If it says a high number, then I have to accept it. I did make a huge pig of myself this week while dealing with my daughter's pneumonia. I felt like my life was stressful, so I ate food to deal with it. That excuse is not good enough to put on pounds.

Tonight I sit here wishing I had a friend to talk to other than myself. I kind of get sick of sharing thoughts with myself. I am not a vain person. You need confidence to be vain, and I lack that quality.

Wandering Mind

My husband asked me tonight what I could imagine myself doing for a living that would make me really satisfied. I quickly thought of hideous things that don't exist anymore, like running a record store. No one even buys records anymore, and somehow I seemed to have lost track and gotten left in a time warp. My husband quickly said that MP3 players would definitely keep me from running a record store. What would I do if I had a choice? Well, I would write songs and do anything that put me around music.

I wish I were someone important. Then I could be anything I wanted. I used to dream about running a dance club, one with all kinds of talent on stage, sort of like an open mic night on Fridays and Saturdays. I often dreamed of a dance club that was cool that was full of people every night. Then thoughts of crime and drug pushers and fights breaking out seemed to cloud my mind on the idea of a public place that I ran. Why does every dream that pops into my silly head have a bad ending? What if I actually ran a club that didn't have someone getting shot outside in the parking lot? It is rare to run a nightclub where some crime doesn't randomly occur.

Sometimes I dream that I am a famous painter with a gallery of art for the world to just walk in and see. I would have hidden cameras everywhere to capture comments about my art. Sometimes I laugh thinking about being a fly on the wall of some place where I know I am the topic of conversation.

Getting back to the matter of dream jobs, I would like to be a singer on stage at a giant coliseum. I would make the crowd go crazy with my songs that reach their deepest thoughts and feelings. Song writing is truly an art, and I believe those who write hits are talented and blessed to be able to do it. It seems that every time I dream of a perfect job, it includes music. If I could work at a record company, that would be totally cool too.

I have always been jealous of movie producers, the way they get the chance to read all kinds of scripts. It must be rewarding to be the person behind a multimillion-dollar movie. Why can't I be someone important like movie producers or rock stars?

I thought that being a soap star might be fun, but the first moment I had to kiss a costar, I would get grossed out and run away. I would not be that great at pretending to be romantically involved on the set of my show. I would be the worst soap star ever. I guess for now acting dreams are not part of my plan.

Where can I go in this world and feel happy? That is the million-dollar question. It seems every job has its yucky moments. When I work as a substitute teacher, other teachers talk to me rudely, especially the older ones. Whenever I come in contact with them in a room, they tell me off somehow, making me hate my job. Most ask me to leave as soon as they see me.

I once was a maid for an entire year of my life. What I learned was that I couldn't clean as fast as others I called lifers. The second thing I learned about myself as a maid was I looked bad in the uniform. Third thing I learned was that most of the maids I worked with stabbed me in the back and stole my towels and bathroom supplies, so they did not have to go downstairs to get more.

I have a personal weakness about myself that keeps me from telling off offensive people. Most of the time I hide my anger well and never show it until I get home, and then it appears to those who never did anything wrong. I call it my work- anger-transference time. I wish that somehow I could express anger at the correct times, but it does not happen. I have delayed anger reactions.

I want a job where I can use my education and my mind. I feel that I earned a degree I cannot use, as if no matter where I apply, people do not choose to hire me. They choose someone else. I have ugly clothes and a look about me that says I am not worth hiring. I need money to buy clothes, and I need a new me. I want to be that pretty girl who applies and gets hired for her looks. Since I am plain Jane in the looks department, I need to come up with a better plan.

I applied for four jobs in the last few days. I hope someone finds me likeable so I can leave the substitute work I am in. I hate my job, every moment of it. I wish I never chose that type of work. One thing is for sure; a job must be compatible with your personality, or it becomes a big giant burden mentally. One thing I know about myself is that I feel obese. My son says that I am three feet wide, side to side. I tested that theory and drew lines with pen on my closet door when no one was looking. It read seventeen inches wide. That is chunky fat, and I really need to start walking on my treadmill.

The sexy new sleek me is waiting for me to exercise. I made big mistakes today and ate Hershey kisses and those cool pink snowballs. I do not think that was part of my diet plan, to eat that crap. I fell off my diet-plan wagon once again. What set me off this time? My husband made me attend yet another boring event with Boy Scouts. It sent me into an eating frenzy when I got home. The kids were so badly behaved at the event that I developed a migraine yelling at them to listen to me. Why is it so hard for me to let them just be young kids?

I tell myself that any job can be something I adapt to. It doesn't seem to be the case with my current job. My current job makes me feel like throwing up. I hate even thinking about going to work tomorrow. I pray daily that God will open up an opportunity for me to start working somewhere I will be happy. I wait patiently for God to answer my prayers. I tell my kids that God can do anything, and I really believe that he can. He will help me lose weight. I just have to be patient.

I need to start over yet again tomorrow with no more eating of chocolate, cheese, or cookies. Tomorrow I will limit myself to healthy veggies and fruits. Tomorrow I will keep up my spirits and believe in myself enough to exercise. My treadmill needs to be plugged in and used from now on. I will make myself dance an hour, making sure I burn extra calories.

If I hold myself responsible for what I eat, maybe then I will be more aware of my caloric intake. I will now start a calorie journal I show my husband daily. Maybe the humiliation of showing him will force me to change. Every day that I lose to overeating is one day I cannot get back.

If I could turn back time, I would go back to when I lost lots of weight and felt better. I would try to keep from gaining weight back. I know in my heart I am a stress eater. I eat when I emotionally cannot handle situations. I had to discipline my kids and found myself eating food for no reason ten minutes later.

I wish I could cook like chefs on TV and feel great while doing it. Guilt always runs through my mind when I use oils and other things for ingredients. I wish I could cook without guilt. When I use meats, I feel guilty and wonder if I am killing myself by consuming more fatty things. I want to be a vegan, but my husband says I don't have the ability to give up things like meat. I do love chicken meals, such as in Chinese foods. Maybe there is a better answer for me than giving up everything.

Cursed Week

Have you ever felt cursed by the world? I feel that way this week. To begin my unlucky trend of a week I called to check on a job I was supposed to do as a substitute teacher. The lady on the other phone stated to me that my four-day job was cancelled completely. That would mean 240 dollars of pay I would not earn. I needed to earn some money because I am in the hole by $700 a month, and I fear losing all that is necessary. The secretary set me up for another job the next day, and I felt some relieved that I would make thirty dollars this week.

Aftercare for my children runs ninety-six dollars a week, so even thirty dollars would mean I was in the hole by sixty-six dollars. I arrived at my job hoping for a half day's work, only to find that the teacher was working. He asked me to leave, because he no longer needed a substitute. I could not believe my cursed week. How can I buy groceries or pay for bills if no one will employ me? Here I am with a bachelor's degree in pre-law, and I cannot find work for even one full day. I definitely need a job that pays well. I wish that all those times I worked hard to make an A in college mattered. I prayed out to God in fear that I would not have to take my kids out of aftercare. The only way I can work all day is if I have someone picking them up after school. I love my children and don't want to work evenings. I look forward to helping with homework and playing Monopoly and video games with them. How can I support my family if no one will hire me?

I set out to apply for many jobs over this past weekend. I feel a sense of anxiety inside because I fear that no one will call me, and if they do, maybe they will dislike me. I do not have one nice outfit to wear to an interview. The clothes I wear to work now are torn and lack hems in the bottom of the shirts. I am embarrassed by the fact that I don't ever look professional.

I was sitting here daydreaming about being rich and famous. I like to imagine winning Publishers Clearing House and everything being great in my life.

My grandma used to love Publishers Clearing House contests. When she died I took over where she left off. I always enter and dream of winning big. My state will have the lottery in a little more than a year. Maybe I will win.

Today I feel that I am cursed because nothing is going the way I need it to. I wanted to work five days straight, but on Monday my daughter was ill, and the week before that, I missed work because I had pneumonia. I need to catch a break.

I got on the scale today and felt that the scale hated me. It went up three pounds, even though I starved myself all day yesterday. I even stopped drinking liquids. I think that was a terrible plan.

Do you know what I would do if I were rich? Get one of those great personal trainers at the gym. It occurred to me last night while I lay in bed that I have no idea how to work out.

I wish that I had work to go to. I would be happy to earn a living this week. A big portion of America is out of work, so I guess I should feel blessed to be employed, at least. Did I mention how much I hate my job? Every day is like that sound of nails on a chalkboard that people dislike. No one treats me like a human. I think even the janitor snubbed me last week, which was very sad.

I have started reading my favorite book again about self-esteem. I have read it three times before, but it inspires me, and I need that book right now. I like to lose myself in a magazine or book to dull the emotions I feel toward my unsuccessful lonely world.

Ball Dropped

Today in the midst of what I thought to be a great Friday, I found out some not-so-positive news. My husband lost his job. This is a second time in less than six months that he will be searching for a new career. The worst part is that I do not have work either. I worry we will not have a roof over our heads. I am afraid to breathe and afraid to move right now. It feels like a ball dropped on me, and I did not catch it. The bad-news ball bounced on my dreams of having a big back yard garden. As I watched my devastated husband walk out to the back yard and take the fence out of the lawn, I could only sigh. What had I done to deserve moving yet again from a place where I felt secure? In nine years I have moved eight times, and honestly, I thought we would stop. I cannot blame my husband for the economical problems going on.

I wish somehow I could help make things better everywhere. I am afraid of not having health insurance, and I wish I could go to a dentist. I need fillings, but that is the furthest from my mind. My husband says we will lose our home and file bankruptcy in exactly nine weeks, so here I am counting down to a very scary place. I am not a stranger to starting over. Material things are not more valuable than those I love. My family is my world, and wherever they are, I will be happy. The pain is from paying bills on time for nine years straight, keeping perfect credit, only to have it all pulled out from underneath me. The ball dropped today as I watched the words come out of his mouth, "I lost my job." He was the breadwinner in our house.

I am fighting off a migraine that has already gotten me sick and made half my face numb. I have to hide my fear from the kids. They thought this home would be a place where they could grow up. We made all those promises to the kids. We bought the acre behind our house a month ago. I am scared of what will happen to us. I fear we will end up living in the car or in some sleazy flea-invested hotel. I pray to God that things look up for my husband and me.

The worst thing about all this is that I feel like I am a bad person and bad wife. How can I make things better? No one will even give me a call back when I apply for jobs. I guess that is what most of Americans feel right now, a sense of desperation about our futures.

Somehow I will make things better for my family. I offered to work nights and weekends while my husband works days. I will go without food and sleep to help fix our sad situation. This turn of events will not break us, and we will survive bankruptcy and loss of our home. I love my family, and I love my country despite all these economic problems.

Speaking of loving my country, I went to my mailbox a few days ago. I found an envelope. It was a U.S. Army Freedom Team salute. It included a thank-you letter and a certificate of thanks for being a soldier's angel to a wonderful soldier named Sundi. I wrote her while she was away in Iraq. My face felt flushed with embarrassment because I felt that I didn't deserve the certificate. Sundi served our country. I cherish her and all soldiers who fight for our freedom and safety. I wrote her because I wanted her to know I was praying for her to come home. Praise God for all things, because she did come home to her son, and I was happy for her safe return.

I had never known another soldier in war, and I felt that before becoming a soldier's angel, I had no idea what pain the soldiers felt from being away from their loved ones. I will always thank my soldier for her sacrifices and what she taught me about being strong. If she could go a long time from her family and friends and still come out okay, then I need to be strong too. If I have to start my life over with my family, I will find a way to be strong inside, just like Sundi, my hero.

My husband will be going on a trip soon. I will go on a fast from food, drinking only tea. I want to fast and pray while he is away on a business trip. I need a miracle to help us. The countdown for his job being gone is nine weeks away, maybe even sooner. I wish I could tell my relatives, but I do not want to worry my mom or dad. They have their own lives, and I don't need to stress either of them out.

I never like worrying my parents, so I will keep this job loss, fore-closure, and bankruptcy future to myself until it is absolutely necessary for me to tell them the grim news. My husband seems unusually calm about it all, but I think he is in shock, just like me. Where will we end up? I wonder if we will be in a soup kitchen somewhere in a shelter. I hope that my children will understand all these changes in their lives. Dear raincoat, I sure could use a rainy day to wear you and feel secure. I think I will put you on for security right now.

I am pretty sure that my ugly raincoat is a security blanket from everything. It covers me like a large tent and gives me a reason to smile sometimes. Often people laugh at my ugly coat, but I feel I need to wear it. I own very few clothes. I don't even have an interview outfit. The clothes I wear to work are missing hems, and coworkers laugh at me for my hideous clothes. When it rains I can cover up my embarrass-ing lack of style for just the day.

I sit here staring at my husband in disbelief that I may very well move out of Arkansas to another state in a little more than two months. We have no savings and nothing in our checking account. We have no way to relocate. I sit here worrying about the future for my children. I hope for their sakes we move somewhere safe. If I could just land a great job, I could help out.

I applied for work today and found that wearing heels that are too high can be a danger in a courthouse. I almost leaped into the air after losing my balance in my shoes. I have never been perfect at going down a double flight of stairs. I am an elevator person, because of my clumsiness. I hoped that the person who took my application did not see me tripping on my way out. First impressions are important.

New Look

I decided to get a hair cut today. It was time. After all, I had unhealthy hair that went all the way down my back, and it looked bad in interviews. I decided that I needed an updated look, because I am in my late thirties and still had a teenager hairdo. I know this to be true, because I teach in a high school every day and have something to compare myself to.

As I stared deeply into the mirror, I wondered if I would really hate myself later for the shoulder-length look. My hair seems to grow slower than before. I got on the Internet and intently studied female professionalism in the workplace. I found that many people wrote of hair being the number-one thing that can keep a person from being hired. I took inventory in my head of what I looked like at my recent interviews. I wore a ponytail pulled back so tight it looked like I had a face lift.

The time for change in me on the outside is now. Today, March 23, 2009, I begin to look more like the smart business mind that I am inside.

Today my husband went on a week-long business trip, and I am home for the week with my children on spring break. The kids will be bored because it is supposed to be raining all week long.

I am taking this week-long opportunity to clean my house and make it wonderful. I want to take pride in the things that I am blessed with. My children are my biggest blessing. I want to make my house as clean as possible to show my gratitude for all that I have.

Sometimes I feel a sense of jealousy of those who seem from the outside to be happy, those people with one hundred best friends all posted on social networks for the entire world to see. I feel jealous of those couples that have all the support in the world when they need a babysitter. I always find myself praying that I will not be jealous of those who have it so very easy. Life has not been easy for me, and I wonder how it is for others with no support system in place.

I love life and I love my kids, and I never regret having them. Sometimes it feels that I wish I could be a more patient person.

I looked in the mirror hoping that my new hairdo, which is now shoulder length, was not a large mistake. I look different now. Suddenly I feel ten years older, I guess because in my mind, I remember all my aunts having shorter hair when they were older.

I find myself lost in thought sometimes. I have found that I do not fit in to normal society. I honestly don't care about things that most do, such as nails, expensive jewelry, and clothes. Some men have called me cheap before, but that is how I think. Things of material value mean very little to me.

Now I see that the person I am and what fits in to a normal society is not the same. As I change my outside to feel more confident, I also need to work on my self-worth on the inside. Every hour that passes by, I feel sickened inside, hoping that I can get through this. Honestly I wait in fear that my husband will come home and say today was his last day at work.

For my new look I went to the clearance section of the store and found the best suits I could find. It was quite a bargain at nine dollars each piece. I knew they were the wrong size, and I am about forty pounds from fitting into the clothes. Still, I am all set to look like I work at a bank. As I stare blankly into the mirror, I say this over and over, that I am strong and smart and worth knowing. Despite a lifetime of questioning everything, I think this is it. I am going to change me for the better.

I made it one day while my husband was away on a trip. I sure feel unhappy that he left me with a spring break vacation week. I am parenting with no help or break the entire week. Nothing new for me; there are never any friends to help out. Thank goodness I am already prepared to be lonely and tired. If my husband loses his job in a few months, we will have no money, no jobs, and definitely a sense of nowhere-land feelings.

Honestly lately I have been turning against those friends or so-called friends who never write or return e-mails. How can anyone consider himself or herself a friend if he or she never seems to be there for you when you need them? You know what? I have downgraded many e-mail friends to just acquaintances I know distantly. I have promised myself that I will no longer try and be friends with those who have refused to write back. What is the use of chasing after people who only take and never give of themselves? I say go away, takers and emotional vampires who write only when they need to be picked up. They never return the favor.

Yes, today I do inventory, and if some man or woman doesn't add to my quality of life, I will refuse to write that person, even one more time. I am freeing my soul from the feelings of rejection. I am definitely not okay with hearing from a so-called friend once a year. Here I am looking at my new hairdo and wondering what I was thinking. I hate it; now it is something I must live with. I have that new-hairdo-regret thing happening.

My day was stressful and terrible today, and I am hoping tomorrow will be much better. I have confidence if I put forth more effort to be positive that even a gloomy rainy day could be pleasant. I am still hoping that the kids will like my new hairdo. I asked my son if I looked better than the day before. He told me honestly that he didn't remember what I looked like before.

I took a funny journey today on one of those social networking websites. I wanted to see if I could find people from my past, and I did. It was weird to see them ten or more years later from when I knew them. I bet if they saw that I had gained ninety pounds they would surely be sick to their stomachs. I don't want to be a chunky person, but I am. I guess obese is not exactly chunky, but a lot bigger. I have one enemy I must fight for weight loss, and that is my stress and my bingeing.

The Interview

I had a job interview today. I felt ready, really confident about myself for once. I wore a business jacket, and my hair was fantastic. I curled it just like I saw on television a couple of days ago. I felt as if I could do anything today. I was on top of the world. I did answer questions all wrong, at times. I am sure that the other applicants will slip a few times too. I found out that I was one of five candidates to get interviewed. Even better was the fact that they would make a decision Friday. I have only one long week to wait it out and see. Who will it be who gets hired, my competition or me?

As I drove to my interview, many fears came across my mind. One fear was that my great hairdo would be ruined because the rain came down like a flash flood as I drove closer and closer to the place. The job that I was interviewing for was one that most people in this town would love to have. I earned a bachelor's degree, and I deserve an opportunity to prove myself. Too many times I have thought that jobs didn't give me the opportunity to use my mind. I knew this job would be what I needed.

As I sat there and listened closely to what both interviewers had to say, I felt a confident. That confidence must have come from God, because I don't remember ever having an ounce of confidence. I started to think about things while they were talking. I wondered what the others would be like in their interviews. Was I going to stand out in their minds?

In the back of my mind I wanted to feel happy and say to myself, "Yes, I do deserve this job." I wanted to beg them to choose me. I wanted to yell, "Hey, please choose me over the other applicants." I didn't think I could handle one more day of mindless substitute teaching.

I know one thing I should have remembered to take, an umbrella or good raincoat on a rainy day. I love wearing raincoats; they make me feel safe and happy. I made the mistake of saying that the job would make me happy, a comment that did not go over very well with the interviewer. I promised my husband before I went to the interview that I would smile. I promised him I would do everything perfectly. I was not perfect at all. That is okay, though it's over, and I am sitting here nervous and waiting for the day to go by. Today is interview day. After today the two men will decide if I am the next secretary. Had I said enough right things for them to remember me? Only they could answer that question.

On my way home, I felt happy and glad it was all over, but now I question some of my crazy answers. I can be over the top at times. It felt like I was too aggressively pushy about using my mind. As I sat listening to them speak, I felt as if I could really work with both men daily. They seemed smart and nice, just like I see myself.

As I sit here talking to God while the rain comes down, I don't feel alone at all. I pray he helps them choose me, if that is where I should be. I did my part. I dressed nicely and told them what I could do, and it is out of my hands now. I am glad that they considered calling me. What an honor to get an interview!

The rain came down as I drove home and my windows began to fog up. I was happy that I had tried to change my life. I know now that I can be classy and I can dress and feel great. Even if I am overweight, I can change things about my exterior self that helps others see who I really am. I discovered that I am the woman who likes business suits. If the company does not hire me, then I am off to apply at a bank.

Whatever they have in mind, I will find out very soon. I will either get that sad letter in the mail that says we chose someone more suited for the job or a call that says we have to see you for a second interview. I own only one suit, so I hope the interview process is fast.

I believe that I will transform my life into something better if I keep trying and get myself out there. The world has not seen what I can do yet.

I loved that the interview questions were not silly. Sometimes job interviewers ask crazy problem-solving questions that I find boring. They were great questions pertaining only to the job itself, which was perfect.

Did I have a successful interview? I think I did, and as I walked away from those two individuals, I felt that they connected with me in some way that would increase the likelihood of my being hired. Still I am afraid to get that call from my husband that says we are moving out of the state. I want to feel secure and able to have roots somewhere. I don't blame my husband for all the economical problems of our country or his job instability. I just want a chance at a great career where I feel useful and capable of being the best worker and person I can be. Life sure has not been easy for me. I haven't had a lot of people to lean on lately, so I want this great job.

I love rainy days, but not when I have an interview. I can think of two specific interviews that went out the door on rainy days. One was a bank teller job. My coat hood had fallen down, all the rain washed my hair flat, and my clothes were dripping all over her chair. I tried to fix the situation, but nothing seemed to sway her looks at my wet clothes and me. Rain can be a bad thing on interview day, especially if you do not own an umbrella.

My second rain interview to go terribly wrong washed out my mascara and made my shirt buttons pop off. I should have gone to a bathroom and looked in the mirror before my video conference interview. I would have noticed my hair was horrible and my makeup was scary. I have learned from experience to bring a mirror to look at, if it rains. The rain did not get me this time, because I ran to my car after the interview and avoided getting messy. My waterproof mascara sure was useful today. I guess it really doesn't run if wet.

I am filled with joy today, even if I do not get the job, because I know that I am someone special. Today is the day that I feel loved by God and by me, and I feel fantastic. Today I am filled with a sense of joy and peace that God placed in my heart. Nothing of this earth can take that from me at this moment in time. I am thankful for this emotion I feel. I hope it lasts a very long time.

Speaking From the Soul

Today is Monday; thank goodness for that. I made a promise to my first-grade son today. I asked him to believe in me, and he said he would. I told him today, Monday the twentieth, I would go on a diet and successfully lose one hundred pounds. He looked at me and said he loved me, no matter what. I kept saying to him, "Do you believe in me?"

He kept saying, "I do, Mommy. I do believe that you can do this." Then he asked me a profound question quickly. He said, "Do *you* believe that you can lose weight this time?"

Thoughts rushed through my head. How could my son see my personality so clearly?

All day long I rushed to think about all the tiny ways I show the kids just how little I believe in myself. It is very important that they think I at least believe in myself.

My husband had a breakdown yesterday, crying and screaming, admitting he wished he was dead all the time. He said that he often hopes not to make it home from work. He hates everything about us right now. I guess I haven't been someone who could ever make him happy. As I stood and heard his depressing words of wished-for suicide, I could only be angry at him. Did he think life was happy or easy for me all these years? I knew that his possible job loss in a couple weeks was making him less strong and more vulnerable to anger and sadness with the kids and me. His death wish was more than I wanted to hear that day.

If I did not feel terrible about myself before, I did at that moment. He said he wished he was dead so he didn't have to feel the way he does around me and the kids. I wish my husband had lots of friends, but he doesn't really try to make friends. If they try to make plans with him, he cancels or never accepts their invitation. Somehow if I were magical, I would change his life and mine.

Do you know what life has taught me about many men? They won't let me leave freely when I say good-bye. Often I have to escape them when they least expect it. That is not love at all. Why do people hold on to relationships that are not good for their soul? I am one of those people. I drive Chris crazy with my depression. I actually feel bad for him, because he married me. It wasn't good for him having to live with me.

I know that change is needed, but I don't feel I have freedom to do anything about it. How do I show the kids I believe in myself, if all we ever hear is that we are bad and that we are not worth living for? I wish I had friends to talk to. I don't have anyone to talk to, because I can't burden my parents with minor things like my happiness. They have problems of their own. If I could say something clearly out loud for the world to hear all at once, I would say, "I Love the lord more than anything." Many might not care that I even said that. Lately I have been saying to my husband that God can do anything. He always looks at me like I am crazy to even speak those words.

Last week while substitute teaching, I was walking to my class. It was a dreaded class with kids I knew would be disciplinary problems. As I walked through the campus, the children yelled out at me. One boy said, "Hey, everyone, look at her fat butt." He gathered fifteen or more people to yell things out at me as I walked by. They were telling me I was a cow. I prayed that God would keep me from cussing or crying; either one could have happened. Luckily I was spared that day, and my emotions and logic took over to protect me. My anger gets me in trouble often.

I knew that the kids were correct in calling me fat. After all, I was 120 pounds over my needed weight. I just expected the eighth and ninth graders to be a lot more polite than they were. I was sad the entire day as I drank water only and didn't touch food. I felt empty inside from the harsh words.

My battle here on earth seems to be with eating and myself. I daydreamed for hours about how nice people would be if I were thin and beautiful. It seems the last year has been hard for me. All those people I thought would e-mail me for support or check up on me to see how I was sometimes disappeared, no matter how much I wrote them. One thing is for sure, that you cannot make people be there for you. They have to put you as a priority. I have learned that I am not anyone's priority.

I refuse to let this destroy me as a person. I will look in the mirror today and heal from all these things that are trying to break my spirit. I love me, and my soul keeps trying and trying to better me. I can lose weight this week. I got on the scale and weighed 213 this morning. I lost two pounds this weekend. I have no idea how I did that, but who really cares? The less I weigh, the better off I will be. My depressing life has been helping me drop weight slowly from 240 pounds.

I watched romantic drama on the television last night. All the actresses are so thin and perfect. I want that to be me one day. I will set my goals high and win at this battle of obesity. I promised my son today that I would believe in myself if he believed in me. I will not let him down this time.

Social Networking

No one ever promises that life will get easier. For me it has just gotten harder and harder. I am married with no friends and no family around me. Some days are just full of hearing the kids fight or my husband yell at the kids. Tomorrow is Mother's Day, and I wonder if the kids will make me some cards or something. Lately my bored mind has been wandering around endlessly on the Internet sites. I joined social networking websites. I wanted to see how easy I could make friends if I tried. I didn't use my real name.

I learned some painful truths. One truth was that my friends who were always too busy to write me a few lines in an e-mail or call me were available hourly on the social networks. I learned that a few of my e-mail friends who write only once every few months were committed to being popular and shallow online. What big thing did I learn? Rejection with this type of social networking is still difficult. I read an article that said the number of people on social networks continues to rise in the millions. Another social network website experience was all too painful for me to see. I realized that my e-mail friends that gave me the cold shoulder were there too. I found family members online sharing even the most detailed parts of their lives, like what they were eating that night.

I made a personal decision tonight that I will find a way to communicate with people that completely avoids using my computer. I will write more letters and I will call more often and visit more in person. The harshest reality about social networking on the Internet is that predators can find an innocent woman's job or her home much easier by just being a friend and watching her every move daily. Many people write that they are leaving on vacations and many say they are going just about anywhere at all. You can tell more about a person by the amount of friends they have collected on the social networking.

Just to be fair, after only a few days of looking without rose-colored glasses at my friends on websites, I realized that watching their thoughts on the public Internet wasn't the same as hearing from them personally.

From this day forward, I will focus on changing how I feel about me. I must say one good thing happened, though. I made friends with one of my favorite singers on a social network site. He listed me as a friend, and I was very excited that someone as talented as he is would do that. Even if I am just a fan, it made me smile.

I want to make friends in person, face to face, from now on. I have no reason to prove how great I am online. I am writing tonight because I feel set free. My addiction to watching others' daily events is gone. I think I am very sick of those three-sentence e-mails that tell me nothing and ask me how I am. When I respond I never hear back from them. Do you know what kind of friends I want? I want friends that call me and spend time with me and also return e-mails with answers to my questions. All these shallow relationships I currently involve myself in feel like an emotional drain.

Tomorrow I will start a new church, and I hope to become renewed spiritually. I feel lost and cannot figure out why all I feel is hate toward life and people and technology. What I have learned from my own experiences is that people are rude to my face, and I can find them posting friendly blurbs on social networking sites only hours later. It is easy for people to be fake, when there are no actual human beings around to see them cursing the world. No one is real anymore, and it has taken its toll on my emotions and feelings.

I had a dream the other day. I was a star on some talk show, like that would ever happen, and the host says to me in a joking way that she has a secret guest on the show. I am afraid at this point in the show because I think she will bring back some hideous person from my past, but then I remember she is classy and would not do that. In my dream she introduces a singer and he plays one of his songs. It was the best dream ever, and I wish it were a premonition. Getting on a talk show would be a difficult task. Lately my addiction to music video websites has grown. I like to look up songs from the 1980s to sing along. I just wish when I was a teenager I had been able to access music videos easily.

I fear sometimes that all this easy access can be truly dangerous for the kids. I worry that my own kids will search things that are inappropriate when I am not standing near the computer. I worry about how to protect my kids from the Internet social scene that is very popular with young students currently.

Vegan

I got on the scale to find that after four months of dieting, I had gone up in weight by quite a lot. I am currently 220, and I am looking at my own death wish, if I don't drop weight soon. My heart is bothering me, and I do not want to die, so here is my solution: to become a vegan. I see those people all the time, and they are thin and healthy. That is my deal with myself. I will become a vegan. I wish I knew how to say it correctly so I did not sound like an idiot. My husband's favorite word when angry is to call people an idiot.

I am on my first day of my vegan diet. No milk-product slipups yet. I am truly addicted to cheese. I was viewing a photo of myself from yesterday's Mother's Day celebration. I looked liked a hideous cow. How can I stand to look at myself anymore? The worst part was today I had a new photo taken when I renewed my license. Now I must be forced to look at my chunky self for four more years.

Don't get me wrong; I like that it was so easy to get my license renewed. The worst part is I wanted to be skinny when I renewed it. There just wasn't time to drop one hundred pounds in a few weeks.

I ate a salad today and did not have cottage cheese, cheese, or meat in it. It felt empty and lonely without that stuff. It felt as if I was some bunny rabbit eating a head of lettuce. How can I do this? How can I give up chicken, tuna, and cheese products? I pray that God gives me some inner strength. This time I must do this for myself and no one else.

My second goal for May 11 is to run on the treadmill and start to get in shape. I want to compete in a 5K one day, and I know I must practice to build up strength to do that. I know I can.

My head is spinning and my headache is making it difficult for me to function, but I have to pretend I am fine. We cannot afford for me to go to the doctor. As I sit hear dreaming about having the perfect job, I wish I had a bag of money. I wish I had money so I could go to the dentist. We have dental insurance that covers only 80%, and I just do not have the other portion. I find myself jealous of all those people with ultra white teeth. I wish I were one of those pretty people.

I have downloaded lots of information on vegan eating and plan to read it all. My other goals for this week are to start learning a new language and write some songs on my guitar. Song writing is so much fun for me, and I feel like there is nothing more fun than writing lyrics.

I heard a country band as I was driving in my car today. That band is one of the best country bands ever. If I had a sound card in my computer, I would listen to videos by that band. I no longer have any way to hear them on the computer, so I just sing their songs by memory.

I plan to be the best vegan I can possibly be. I may call myself a vegetarian, because it is easier for me to pronounce. A lot of celebrities go on strict diets to stay trim. I hope this type of eating helps me in the long run. I measured myself last night and found that I was as fat as I had ever been. My lower abdominal area was fifty-two inches. No wonder I am knocking down my kids when I run into them in doorways. My boy is always saying to me, "Mommy, you sent me flying across the room." If my butt hits him while we are walking through a doorway, he goes flying off like a volleyball sometimes. He is just a little forty-four-pound child.

As I sat eating food this morning, my son says to me that he would not know what to think if I were skinny. He said that I have always been fat as long as he was alive. He is right about that. I have always been an obese mommy to him. I believe in my heart I can change.

The Tornado

It was a Friday in June and I got a text message from my dear husband. He stated that his boss moved him to a safer place in the building because a tornado siren went off in his town. The place he works is about twenty-five minutes away. As I read his text message, my power went off. I wondered why my power was gone, because just moments before, we had bright sunshine.

I ran to the window to see what in the world was going on outside that might turn out my power. What I saw next put fear in me. I saw a tornado coming right for the house. I only had seconds to grab both kids and hide somewhere that had no glass windows. I was afraid that it was going to flatten the house. I didn't know if we would survive. Fear was going through my mind of just how mean I was to God the day before. Was this my payment for yelling out loud? I had little faith in society and did not care anymore about anything.

I had read once in the Bible that God disciplines his children. Was I going to be flattened by a twister because I was acting in a bad way toward God?

I sat in fear as the twister circled my house and lifted the top off my roof above my head only to slam it back down where it was to begin with. My children screamed out and cried. Neither knew if we would survive. My little girl is autistic and was becoming very difficult to calm down. She started rocking back and forth, and my son leaped over her head and said, "Don't worry; I will protect you, little sister." I was proud of my son, only seven years old. What a brave person he is becoming! He is such a good kid.

After the roof dropped down where it was to begin with, I could tell the tornado had left the area. I looked outside at all the debris of chopped tree limbs. The phone rang, I answered it, and it was my husband. I was glad to know that he called the electric company for me. Five hours later, the power returned and the kids were able to relax again. All I could do was pray in thanks for the safety of my children and myself. I was glad my husband was safe too, at his job.

I still find myself wondering why the tornado went completely around my home. It felt like angels were surrounding my house. I don't question things like that, and I will always be thankful we made it through that creepy scary tornado day. I always thought that Kansas was the only place to see so many tornados. That was all before I moved to Arkansas, where tornados are a regular occurrence.

It has been dry lately, and I have not had a chance to wear my raincoat, but I think of it often. It always makes me feel skinny and happy. My ugly raincoat gets laughed at, and it has holey pockets now. My keys fall out of the pockets, but it is still my security blanket. I feel like I can do anything with it on. I will put it on today to smile.

My weight is still going up and my migraines are taking over my life almost weekly now. Sometimes I wonder if I will wake up not knowing who I am when I become so sick from migraines. The tornado occurrence took my mind off the pain in my head for a moment.

I had prescription medicine on which I deliberately doubled the dose today, to fight off the pain. It helped slightly, but I am not sure how safe it was.

My current weight after the tornado is 218. That is sickening and may be my big source of headaches. I am supposed to take high blood pressure medicine but haven't, since I have no money to go to the doctor or buy medicine. I just live with high blood pressure and headaches. I wish my life would pick up some.

Separating Thoughts

Here I am lost and fat as ever. I got on the scale only to find I had gained six pounds from yesterday to today. What the crap is that all about? I didn't eat much, and I feel like I am on a sinking ship at this point. What will I do if this failed dieting takes me to 250 then 300? Why can't I have my own personal trainer living with me? I know she could help me out here. Oh, that's right; you need money for a trainer.

Today I had some time to rethink that judgment call I had on social networking. I had no idea where to begin, since I decided that this time online social networking would pertain only to my real personality. Who in the world am I, anyway? Truly and honestly, a songwriter and singer is who I really am inside. Even though years have gone by, my soul is alive with music. I decided that those I would add on my music web page were musicians and famous singers from any time I could remember. It didn't take long before many friends were listed on my special space of that social networking site.

I find myself feeling more alive and excited since joining. I found that I feel connected to all friends online, even complete strangers. I read their blogs and messages they send out daily and feel as if I know a little about them. It is very ironic that a skeptic like me would ever fall so fast for spending time on a social networking site, but I will admit

I am addicted to going there. I have only singers and musician friends and go listen to their music every time I get the chance to be online. True, I could listen to them on an MP3 player, but I like reading their daily comments and activities. I even write to my favorite singers often.

Today, as my children splashed around in the pool having the greatest time, I stood melting in jeans and a hot T-shirt. I don't own a swimsuit, and even if I did, it would traumatize the neighbors to see a giant size-twenty-eight woman prancing around the yard like I was in one of those 1980s rap videos for big-butt women.

Today I analyzed just how much pain I am in personally from being obese. Sickened by the thoughts of dying of a heart attack, I tried to find reasons to start my starvation diet the very next day. I made a list in my head of all my addictions that I cannot seem to fight. One very bad addiction is eating cheese. That must be one of the worst things to eat when you're already 120 pounds overweight. I pray in my heart that I can find my true self sometime soon. When I look at how my weight is hurting my life and my happiness in every way, I can't understand why I am still fat. I need to pray about strength for dieting.

Here is my new list for changing my life. I know you're ready to slap me at this point, because I have started over and over on this idea that I deserve to be thin. Tomorrow I will not drink more than one soft drink in a day, even though I really want to. Tomorrow I will get on the treadmill, even if I feel I am dying of an asthma attack. I will not snack between lunch and supper. I have made a very important decision that I am sticking to. If I break one of my rules, I will eat a chocolate laxative. I know that sounds sick to say. I want to get a bad memory in my head of making a diet mistake. I am determined to be a skinny hot person. This has to happen. I can't be that embarrassing fat mom all the kids laugh at when I drop my children off at school. I lived that experience last year, and I can't deal with it again.

I have started writing songs again, and it feels fantastic to be real and true to my heart. I had dreams of being pretty and less trashy looking. Right now I wear men's T-shirts because I can't find clothes that fit me. I am so jealous of fit, beautiful people. I shouldn't hold a grudge when many of them work out and deserve to be happy. I often try to blame my husband for my unhappiness. I am accepting the responsibility now for my own mess. It is time to clean up the mess in my mind that makes me eat. The person I want to be is employed and thin and laughs often.

I want to be glamorous like Hollywood stars. They always look perfect on TV. I wish I looked sexy like that. I cannot be anyone more than myself, so I have to focus on changing.

Sometimes when I walk by my mirror, I find that I hate me. I hate the size of my body and wonder how I could allow this to happen. I started praying for miracles from God that I would wake up 120 pounds thinner. It's time I take charge of my own life and lose this weight that taunts me daily. Dear raincoat, I haven't been able to wear you in weeks, since it never rains anymore. I miss wearing you to feel safe. I miss wearing you over my fat that everyone sees. I don't care anymore that people laugh when I wear you. You help me feel skinny. I miss you. I will dig you out of the closet and wear you a few days. I am so sorry I put you in the closet away from me. You have been my real friend. You never let me down, raincoat.

Summertime Blues

Why is it so miserable right now? I feel like a melting ice cream every time I go out with the kids to play in the backyard. You would think since the body is made up of water that I would have lost a few pounds by now. Last week alone I ate only one meal a day for five days. I got on the stupid scale only to find that I was still 216. I am a big balloon cow. The wind hasn't been blowing at all, and when the sun is out, I feel like one of those cactus plants in the desert. I feel as if I can't breathe when it's summertime. I find myself wondering what all the dragonflies and birds are thinking about.

I have two birds that visit me daily. I named the red one Henry. He always sits on the top of the kids' slide and eats birdseed. I know he has seen me looking at him eat. Henry the red bird seems like he is smiling all the time. I know they have beaks and can't smile, but somehow I know this bird is smiling at me. Maybe I have spent entirely too much time alone and the bird is not thinking at all.

I have spent a great many months—actually years—watching my three favorite crows, and they speak to me, not in a verbal way, but one that I understand. They fly a certain way when a storm is coming. They call out to each other various ways, and somehow I understand them. I feel connected to nature and trees, along with birds. I always tell Chris a storm is coming when I see the trees and the birds.

Owls always frighten me, for some reason. There was a large white owl that was watching outside my son's window for a week. I did many things to try to scare him off, because he was making sounds that freaked out my son. The bird was just staring at my house. I never knew where he went, because one day he was gone. Even when I was a little girl, owls scared me. I think their size is frightening.

Summer has taken a toll on me. I feel like I haven't slept in months. The last time I felt rested was when school was in session. Now we are four days from school being back in session. I wonder if these summertime blues will go away. As the leaves start to fall, maybe I will find my way back to happy feelings.

Finding a Rainbow of Happiness

Sometimes I think about my past and wonder why I ever invested deep heartache in shallow friends or relationships. Here I am age thirty-nine. I am definitely ready to be free of the heavy burdens I placed on myself all the previous years. This year I will create music. This year I will be kind to those who deserve it. I will stop hoping that some people will be my friends and just let them go for good.

This year I will find my rainbow of happiness. So what if I have no one to talk to in my home right now? I am in search of others who need me as much as I need them. Today I joined a new social network online. Okay, maybe I used a cartoon as my picture after using a guitar photo. I looked for people I knew in high school and then those I really loved and adored in my past. I found that cousins were everywhere. What a delight to know that they would actually talk to me online! It was a real blessing to discover.

What started my change for the better was truly the act of one man, a blues singer in Australia. His name is Horace Bevan. One day online I said to him, "Today is my birthday," and he said, "I will send you my CD all the way from Australia." I thought he must truly be kidding. Sure enough, two weeks later, my package arrived. It contained fantastic blues songs, and I couldn't believe some stranger would show me a little kindness. What a true blessing it was to know that the world really has kind people in it. He was nice to me even though I was a stranger.

I decided after Horace sent me a CD for my birthday that I would learn to do kind things for others as well, pay it forward. After I joined the social network website, I began to feel like my life was whole again. I can talk to all these fantastic friends daily by e-mail or just posting on their walls, if I want. It opened my world up to people. My closed, lonely world changed forever in just a few days.

My husband was offered a new job today. We celebrated by sharing a Snickers bar. I know most couples would go out to a nice restaurant. We cannot do that, because we are broke. We can't afford food, water, or milk.

I am out of shampoo, so I look like one of those people who conserves water for a month. I looked hideous when going to the kids' school today with my dirty hair. I wish I had shampoo, and I wish I had socks without holes in them. I wish I had clothes that didn't plain out embarrass me. Sometimes I look at others and see that they get their nails and hair done weekly. Can't they see how much pain I am in just being plain? Life to me and my family isn't about vanity; it's about survival. We ate the worst-tasting food for supper, because I couldn't afford meat. Luckily our wonderful new neighbors invited us to a meal at their home on Labor Day. They had no idea we don't have anything in the fridge or freezer. Thank goodness they didn't ask us to bring anything. We have a total of two dollars in the bank and fifteen bills that went unpaid this month. I wonder if my phone will be turned off, along with power. I didn't even pay the water bill this month.

My friends online can't see that my world at home isn't happy. I am glad for that, because at least I can build them up and make them smile. Praise the Lord, my husband got hired at a new job. Now we won't have to live in the van like Chris has said we would have to. I am excited about that.

I made a decision to start being happy again. I have gone off my anti-depression medication for good. I have to break myself of it, because we can no longer afford for me to have it each day. I will deal with these horrible mood swings secretly without my husband knowing. When I burst out in tears for no reason, I will make sure to be hidden away. All I want to do is find a way to be strong for the family and not burden them with my torturous mind and sadness that I suffer daily.

Finding my rainbow is what I have in mind now. My first step is to start writing my first song for my album. I am searching my heart now to decide what kind of music I am really about. I have evolved into a new person, these past few years. The rocker that I once was seems to creep out in my songs at times, though. I was trying to write a song for someone recently, and for some reason that rock personality in me kept appearing.

I want to be free to be myself, so I have started being honest with my relatives about the fact that I sing and write songs. I hid it for years, because people think at times that is silly to dream about this type of career.

I came to terms with it one day that music and songwriting are all I have ever cared about and known to be true to me. If I do other things, I am not as comfortable as when I write music and songs.

My previous hatred of social networking was completely wrong and misunderstood. Although I miss personal interaction with people, I cherish the thought that I can be on the minds of those I missed for twenty years. Here I am being me online. Welcome to the new and improved Lorrena Bishop.

Dearest raincoat, I needed you today to protect me from a crazy storm, but you were at my house on a hanger. Somehow when I wear you, raincoat, everything is better. I don't care if your pockets have holes and I lose stuff. You're always there for me, raincoat.

I decided to be a Daisy Scout leader for my daughter's troop. I am very afraid that I won't know what I am doing, especially during cookie-sale day. I pray that I can figure out how to be a good leader for those precious children. Daisy Scouts is all that Hannah talks about, and she can't wait to earn her little daisy petals. Life is really like that; we set new goals for ourselves like Daisy Scouts. Later on in life, it's about being great in sports or graduating from college and then finding the perfect career. All this begins with dreams that you had as a child. We have dreams to be someone successful. I remember dreaming at age nine that I would grow up to sing on television music variety shows. Let's face it; the shows were as different as night and day, but they had one thing in common, which was talented musicians and singers.

Help me Breathe

I am feeling lost today. Like most Americans, I am broke and unable to pay my bills. For the last nine years, I paid every bill on time, and then something went wrong. Everything started piling up, and for some reason we have no gas money and no grocery money. My husband drives a vehicle that doesn't have safe brakes on it, and we can't spare money for new brakes. I worry about his safety all the time. I promised my family I would be in to visit them for Christmas, but I have no idea if we can afford the gasoline to travel there.

I pray more than I ever did before. I keep hoping someone will call me for a job interview. Why doesn't my bachelor's degree get me a job at fast-food places or a motel? I offered to do maid work, and they just never call me.

Lately I have been online watching people share on an Internet service. It's been great for me, because it makes me feel like I am not alone. I can't tell anyone that I speak to online that nothing feels right in my life. I don't want to tell them that everything feels painful to deal with right now.

I wish I could wake up tomorrow and have some sweepstakes representative come to my door and say, "You're the next big winner, Lorrena." I would cry and jump up and down. I would be saying, "Thank you,

Jesus." I think I have entered more than seventy-five times this year alone. It makes you wonder why they send me so many in a year.

October will be here soon, and I am very ready for fall weather. The wind started blowing today. I could feel the breeze on my face, and I felt a sense of freedom by just being outside.

I am sitting here looking at my bills knowing that I can't pay them. How I wish a big bag of money would fall out of the sky and land at my feet for me to pay my power bill and my phone bill. That is being unrealistic to dream of money falling out of the sky like manna from heaven. Not paying my bills makes me feel terrible. I already dress like I live in a Dumpster. Most of my clothes have holes in them. I have very little to wear.

No one ever offers to help me with chores or cleaning. My life with the children is pretty hard at times. Both kids have emotional problems from autism, and it's difficult being a maid, accountant, personal assistant, cook, and everything else all alone. Those who constantly have support from family have no idea what life must be like for others or me. It's difficult and makes a person strong because there is no one to rely on, ever. My child is eight years old and has never had a babysitter or ever stayed with grandparents for any reason. I can tell you it has taken its toll on my husband and me never to go out or enjoy one day of our lives. It has always been parenting and chores for me, with no laughter. Girl's night out for women is only a distant dream for me. I can live vicariously through those I know who do live it up constantly.

I don't wish on others whatever it was that I did to deserve the emptiness I live every day. I like to dream about being happy sometimes. I try my best not to show my pain to others in e-mails. There is no use to burden the world with my problems. I talk to God about everything. Despite all that I live through, I know he can hear me up there in heaven. I know in my soul God answers prayers in his own time. I just wish I had patience to wait for him to help me. I wish I could be a better Christian.

As I type this note to you, Raincoat Diary, I want you to know that even with the hardships, I would never trade my life. I can't imagine not being a parent to my little boy and girl. They are everything to me. You gave me two blessings from heaven named Hannah and Luke. I am thankful to you, God, for my loving children. I am sorry that I complain all the time about weight problems. I know that I should be holding my hands in the air thanking you for giving me so much love. I am loved by my children; this I know.

Finding Friends

Dear raincoat, my life is changing. I can feel my heart beating more, and I can feel my soul waking up. I found some people from my past that I loved dearly. I was searching on one of those social networking websites. I realized that love for some people never dies. The things that you saw in them twenty years ago seem to still be there. What I mean is that personality traits that seemed compatible to mine are there. Some people will always be friends for life.

I find myself writing e-mails and letters just out of pure excitement of finding my friends. I guess there is this small fear that life pulled us apart and it could do it again. I am happy about the fact that I found lost friends. Who would have guessed that social networking would be something that I enjoyed instead of feared?

I was thinking lately since it's getting colder that I might not be able to wear you much this winter. I know you have been there for me all these years. I need some warmth. One lady at the elementary school made fun of how ugly my raincoat was. She said, "It doesn't hold out water when it rains." She is right, but that doesn't stop me from wearing you as much as possible. I found a beautiful raincoat at the store and couldn't afford it. It was baby blue in color, and somehow it made me happy just looking at it. I wondered what it must be like for people to shop for clothes when they want. I need clothes but can't even consider thinking about buying them.

My son wears size 4T pajamas and needs size seven. There are holes in the knees of his pajamas and holes in his socks, and I feel terrible because no matter what I do, I don't ever have enough money past bills to buy clothes for the kids.

A paper came home from school the other day. It instantly made me cry. It was a letter asking if we knew any children who needed clothes for Christmas from the local ministries that give to the poor. I felt ashamed because my children need so much. I am too embarrassed to ask for help from anyone.

I live in a really nice home and drive a reliable car and shouldn't ever need to ask for stuff like food and clothes, but the truth is we struggle every day. I am out of medicine and won't tell Chris, because he would feel terrible because he can't buy me more.

I started working on writing songs again lately. I wrote one that I am pretty excited about. That is truly who I am on the inside, a song-writer. I love to write songs for people and bands. I love to sing songs that I wrote. I believe songwriting is second nature to me.

The weather is colder now, because it is two weeks from Halloween. I was supposed to be perfectly skinny by now. After all, I started my journey January 1. I let anger and life get in my way of focusing on weight loss. I feel like I am losing this battle with myself physically. I have something terribly wrong with my legs and can't walk well. Sometimes it feels like I am going crippled. I can't afford a doctor, so I never go get x-rays. My legs just don't want to move when I walk.

Today is October 20, 2009 and I like the twentieth because I was born on July 20. To me this means lucky moments in the day. I like when each month is on the twentieth.

I am making a promise to myself today. I promise to let go of my sadness and focus only on the positive things in my life. I promise to eat healthy and work out daily. I have only one life, and I need to start looking at it that way. I love me. Not in a vain way, but in my heart, I love my mind and my soul and want to be a whole person who is thin and healthy.

Mowing

Our lawn mower died, and I needed to mow my hideously tall lawn, so I got out the push mower. I had no idea how difficult it would be to mow two acres. I started pushing, and it seemed that the mower got heavier and heavier. Every hour got hotter and hotter when the sun started shining. I told myself, "You can do this. You can mow the lawn, and it will be so much better to look at." Anyway, by the third hour, I realized that I needed to stop. I had a migraine. I seem to be allergic to grass at times. Today was one of those days.

As people drove by me watching me slowly push the mower, I imagined them laughing at me. I bet they wondered why I was pushing the mower when we own a riding one. I laughed, thinking about how I don't know how to use a weed eater. If I did, I would go all over the land fixing tall weeds. I honestly don't know how to use one. Sometimes I noticed when people work outside compared to inside. They seem more confident. I think sun exposure makes people feel better. My husband often complains that being in the office can be hard when there is no sunlight to be found. He had jobs where he had no windows to look out.

A Completely New Year

Dear Raincoat Diary, I can't believe it is already January 18, 2010. Here I am 216 pounds and fat as a freaking cow. How did I end up the same weight after a year of fighting myself on paper? I realized something about my true personality during my holiday, and even now. I am never comfortable, ever. I am not comfortable walking near people or even around my kids. I feel fat and unworthy of even being seen by humans.

I have a wonderful friend, Jeannie. She keeps asking to meet with me for lunch. I am afraid if I meet with her, she will notice how fat I have become and not want to be my friend anymore. It's silly to think that way. How would I really know what she is thinking? I don't feel comfortable going to the school and seeing teachers. All the teachers are pretty and skinny and don't understand my complex of obesity.

Sometimes I look out the window and I watch dogs run by and birds fly by. All these animals seem free and uncluttered with guilt complexes, unlike humans. I wish I could wake up free from my own thoughts and fears that keep me still. I would like to wake up tomorrow as someone new and happy.

I came up with an idea lately that I want to try. I want to say to myself over and over, "I am skinny," maybe 500 times, and then see if I change my eating habits in anyway. I know it sounds like a useless idea, but what if it worked?

I started studying fashion magazines, staring at the models. I can see every bone, and their faces look like they lack life. Why can't I be skinny like super models in magazines? Forget the fact they are super tall and I am short.

As I sat endlessly looking at page after page of fashion models without smiles, I started to wonder if one piece of lettuce was their choice of a meal. I wondered if they had great genetics and ate burgers at fast food restaurants. Only the models themselves could answer that question for me.

Sometimes—well, mostly all the time—friends or family members will throw hints at me, even when I don't want them. They give me diet tips when I didn't even bring up weight loss. Most people can't help talking about exercise and eating tips when they see my giant butt. I am fat, and I am aware that everyone sees it.

Being in Love

I have been thinking a lot lately about being in love. I started watching all kinds of shows on TV to observe behavior of what Hollywood says love is. Sometimes I think love means sex only, and that is all that seems to be there. Sometimes I feel that love is about companionship and having someone fix things that go wrong and be there when you need him or her. The alternative is being alone. Being alone is great, but I never seem to be alone. I can't remember a time in my life since I was fourteen years old that I didn't have a man there for me.

I see that one problem I may have in my life was proving that I could be strong enough to live by myself without the strength of a man. I can't say that they all supported me financially, because some stole from me. Sometimes money would come up missing from my drawer. Sometimes my bank account got emptied out. Looking back now, I realize that if I had just taken a single route in my life, I would have so much more saved up and so many other ways to cope. Instead I am a weak link. I am a link in a chain of events that keep occurring. I wonder if my children see how codependent I seem to be.

Back to the subject at hand. What on earth does being in love really feel like? Is it a feeling inside your stomach of joy? Is it an endless need to be with the other person? I can tell you from being married ten years that everything changes. My husband and I didn't even get along when we dated. We fought like cats and dogs. He said he lowered his standards to date me, and I believed him. I should have smacked him in the face for saying it, but I am not the violent type. He can't live it down. I never let him. I hate that I remind him of that comment over and over. To him I was a big fat cow, and in his mind he did lower his standards to date me. I don't feel angry anymore about those words. I have said some pretty rude things in my life too.

Those who have loved for years and years must have a secret of love that they need to share with us lost souls. What was it that kept them going inside? How rare is it to find a soul mate, or is that term one that should never be used? I am inclined to believe that we can love many, and there is more than one compatible partner for us all. Things to avoid when finding true love include someone still going through divorce. Avoid someone who is grieving the loss of a spouse to death or jail time. Believe me, if that spouse gets out of the slammer, you're toast for having taken his or her place for a few months or years. The men going through divorce constantly compare you to the ex they miss and hate. If you do something on a date that reminds them of the ex-wife, they turn on you and decide you're not right for them. Trust me, run away fast from men going through divorce. They simply are not ready to commit or treat you right. They haven't finished healing yet.

Here I am. It's now June 13, 2010. I still weigh about 215 pounds, and I wonder if I will ever be thin. I started going through an angry phase in my life. My sister died of cancer just a month ago, and I haven't been able to deal with that well. I miss her and wish I could hear her voice again. I am angry that she is gone so young, and I am angry that I still can't get out of debt. I have been applying for work for a while now, with no calls coming in.

There is an oil spill taking over the Gulf, and I watch the news wondering what will happen to the beaches and the economy.

We went to church today. It was a new place. I felt like I couldn't breathe. It was full of mostly nice, friendly souls. I actually liked them. The whole time I wanted to run out the door, like a storm was inside my head or heart. I didn't feel like a good enough person to sit with all the people who viewed the world as a good place. All I feel inside is a storm of anger. It has taken over my life.

I felt safe around these people at that the church I visited. They were polite and nice, two things I am not used to being around. I should return to that church.

After the Anti-depression Meds

I made a personal decision to go off of my anti-depression medicine. It was time for me to start on anti-seizure medication, but I didn't want to put more in my body. I quit cold turkey. My life started to unravel at my feet.

The first day off the med seemed okay. I was getting worse by day two withdrawal from meds. I wanted to shoot stuff, run over anything in my way, and also hit everyone with a bat. Time seemed to stop as I went through a private hell.

Three weeks later I have suffered all the symptoms you can think of from withdrawal. I get it why people go to rehab to change their ways. I pushed my way through the bad days. I am now anti-depression-med free, with no more side effects. I pray, giving thanks to God for giving me strength when I needed it most. My weight dropped to 204 when I went off the medication. I am happy about that.

I have all this pressure to lose weight. My husband is always telling me that I need to lose weight. I know he is right, but exercise and starving aren't working out for me. I am now working out to Tae Bo videos. I have found that it helps me feel great daily. I love doing Tae Bo. I am exercising three times a day, and still I am not losing any weight.

True Love

Dearest raincoat, I am here again wondering how my life is going to change if I am completely dependent on my husband financially. It scares me because I have no choice in the matter. We live where he works, and nothing ever changes for me.

I started dreaming constantly about a true love that waits for me. He is beautiful inside and out. He is a lover and friend and the greatest man I have ever known. My true love understands my needs and takes care of me. He waits to save me from the depths of my bored life. My true love enjoys talking to me and listening to me.

I have spent a lifetime not depending on others. I trust only myself, and for good reason. My bored mind takes me back to dreams of my true love. He waits to hold me and love me and tell me that he believes in everything I dream of. This is how I make it through my days and nights. I live in dream world of perfection.

Sometimes when go to get kids at school, I look into the eyes of moms walking by my car. I see sadness. I can tell they had dreams too, before parenting made those dreams invisible. If I had one day when I could live and feel joy doing what I love, I would be singing in some club with a fantastic band playing. I would sing until I had no voice at all. But this dream, dear raincoat, is far from what I live every day. My life is dull and lonely and sad.

If my heart could control every situation and change that which is just not right, then all would be well in the world for me. I would matter, and I would smile even in the darkest of days. Do you know what I lack? Trust for everyone I know. I wish I had it, but cynical ways follow after people let you down over and over.

I wish just once in my life I could know anyone wanted to know me. I wish I had friends I could trust and talk to. There is my British friend who I have known since I was nineteen years old. I can't imagine life without his friendship. He is so important to me. He lives so far away that I never get to laugh and visit him in person.

Sometimes people never know what they mean to me, because I keep it all a secret. We lost track of each other, only to find each other on an online website. How happy I was to find him again. I love him as a soul and a friend. He doesn't ever have negative things to say to me, but encouragement. Stephen is truly my friend, and I am lucky to have found him again after all this time. He finds ways to build me up and remind me of what good qualities I have to offer the world. I cherish him always.

I think the reason Stephen and I like being friends is that we both love music so much. He always talks about British bands he loves. My favorite band of all time is Def Leppard, and the members are from England. He loves Duran Duran. I like them a lot too. Stephen tells me about his travels around the world, and I always learn so much, because I haven't been anywhere. I don't even go on vacations in my own state.

I get a sense of acceptance from my friend Stephen, no matter what I look like. I can tell he doesn't care what I look like; we are friends, and that is all that matters to us both. Stephen is special and unlike anyone else I have ever known. I promised him we would meet one day if we get the chance. I hope that we do meet up. I imagine we would laugh and talk for hours and hours. He always has so much to say about his running. He loves to run.

I think that Stephen makes the world a better place by just being in it. I have never told him so, but I think it often. His soul is kind and trusting and great. He adores his family and is always respectful when talking of them. I wish that I could be more balanced and kind to others, like Stephen is. He is a good person, and I wish I were more like him. I tell him secrets that I don't tell others, and he always listens without judging me. That is the mark of true friendship.

I thank God for Stephen's friendship all the time. It is very good for me to know he is out there. I smile when he sends me an e-mail.

The Scale Again

Raincoat, it has been a while since I told you what I weigh. I avoided it, because the scale did a number on me. I got on one Saturday only to find my weight had spiked again. A feeling of failure came over me. I was 230. I can't believe that stupid scale. Is this weight trying to keep me from feeling happy ever? Yes, friend, I had dreams of being under a hundred pounds, and started doing Tae Bo and yoga with new videos I got, except here I am back at that fat weight. How could someone as short as me be that fat? God help me help myself here.

I have made a decision to join a gym. The question is how do I get my husband to want to join too? I know what to do. I will make him sick by bending over constantly and letting him see my butt. He hates me being fat.

Raincoat, I did what I told you I would do, and it worked. My husband thinks he needs to join a gym. To my advantage, his chair broke at work, and now he feels compelled to find a gym for health and fitness. This is great for me. I can now join dance and other classes to be fit.

My husband took me to the gym for a tour, and I wanted to leave instantly. Everyone was looking at me. I am hideous. They all looked perfect and skinny and happy. Fit people are happy people. Anyway, I made plans to go to kickboxing class, and I really hope I have the nerve to walk in the door and do it. Doing things for the first time has always made me very nervous.

The day came when I had to go to kickboxing class. It was difficult doing all the pushups and sit-ups and running. I looked around the gym class, and everyone was perfect looking. I was dressed badly, and they had the coolest clothes. I don't have nice things.

All the exercising seemed foreign to my TV-watching self. On the other hand, walking out of that gym, I gained something I never had before, a sense of self. I worked out for one hour with kickboxing boot camp. My stomach muscles are torn up and I can hardly walk, but I am determined to make this the beginning of change for me.

Two days later, my stomach muscles are torn so badly from kickboxing class that I can't get out of my chair. I can't move much without wanting to cry. My legs hurt badly, but deep down I want to go back to that class and prove to myself that I didn't break.

I have started reading a new self-esteem book. This book inspires me to believe in myself and make things happen by believing they will, to begin with. I want to make my life a better place, and that process starts with being skinny and healthy. My snack is oranges now, when it used to be Snickers bars.

Changing my Mind and Heart

I woke this morning with a new sense of me. No longer will I get on the scale and define myself as a weight. I am someone of value, and I don't need a man to tell me I am beautiful. From today on I will live for God, for my children, and for myself. I don't want to look good enough for anyone. What good is it if you end up with some self-absorbed vain man who would dump you the first time you gained the old weight back?

Today I am changing my life. Raincoat, I don't need to be perfect anymore. I need to be happy, so I am making a long list of things in my life that make me very happy.

All I really want is to be successful and loved and to love others. Raincoat, it's time I stop crying about things I have no control over and start living. Tomorrow is the beginning of my new attitude and life. I will forgive others when I can and forgive myself too.

What I want and what I need from this life are not out of reach, and I know that if I try really hard, I can succeed. Weakness will no longer keep me from feeling great. I don't need validation, just inspiration. I can be anything I want in this life, beginning with happy. I will take the time to smile every day and live out each day with wonder. I see now that when I started this diary, I didn't believe in happy endings.

Now happy endings are all I can imagine coming true. It's time to throw you away, ugly raincoat that I have worn all these years. It's time to move on and wear other things. Change is good. Thanks for covering me up when I had no confidence to walk into stores. You were a true friend to me. I won't forget you.

I believe inside my mind is someone great, someone ready to help, love, and be there for everyone. I pray for strangers and protect those I love. I am special, and I am worth knowing. It's time I stop trying to prove it to anyone else.

When I wake tomorrow, I am going to sign up for exercise classes. I am ready to face myself, the thing that has been my worst enemy all along. Self-doubts and fears have held me captive for too long. I will wake with a new sense of me tomorrow. I am pretty. I am kind. I am God's child, and I don't need the world. I need God to help me through, step by step. I will talk to God for answers from this day forward. He is the one I should have put all my love into. I am back on the right path.

Job Searching

I never could find a job that I liked, throughout my life. Every job bored me or got on my nerves. I always get a perverted boss who sleeps with young girls and treats everyone else like crap. Being overweight and average looking, I could never get the job luck of the attractive girls, when good-looking men treat you better because they want you. That is how it goes sometimes.

I randomly go about my life knowing that others are going to be rude to me because of my looks.

Today I applied for a job online as a journalist. Maybe I can keep my looks hidden long enough to make a splash in the world. I wrote an article on why women stay in a relationship. I thought it was great material. I wait to see if the newspaper will like it or not.

If I could choose the perfect job, it would be to write songs all day every day for a living. I love writing songs.

I got on the scale today, raincoat. I weighed 200 pounds. Now to most women, that would be horrible. For me it is a good thing. I am on my way back down to a healthier weight. I do feel that life is going to get better. I have decided to limit my intake to 500 calories a day. I feel in my heart that I will fight and win this battle with fat. By my birthday I plan to be ninety pounds. That is 110 pounds less than I weigh now. I believe that I have the power within me to be skinny and healthy.

Today I weighed 198. I can tell the universe is going in my direction. I can tell that what I need and want for myself is going to happen. I have been praying to God for strength with dieting. I am so happy inside my heart right now. I want to get out of the 190s and move as far away from 200 as I can. No one knows the anguish, being fat causes me. For me it's meant not being able to love anyone at all.

I read a magazine today with many sexy stars in it. They all had perfect bodies, and I dreamed about what I wanted for myself. I think I am going to dye my hair blond and become much more fun. I see myself skinny wearing sundresses a lot and having blond hair. I think change is what I need right now. I have been boring my whole life. I need something new. New looks, new body, and definitely plastic surgery, when all the weight is gone.

I am at the beginning of my race. I have just begun, and I plan to go all the way with my weight loss. By July 20, I will weigh ninety pounds.

There is only one week left in this month. I had all these goals to be stronger and better than before. Tomorrow I plan to take a power pump class at the gym. The class is very hard and full of weights and stepping. I fear that I will be the only fat girl in the class, but on the other hand, I see myself being successful at it. They offer this class three days a week. Watch me do this for once in my life. I can and will take this class.

I starved myself today only about 400 calories total. Yesterday I had the same low number of calories. I know it was wrong, but my determination to be thin has started to take over my world. The person that I will become is ninety pounds. She is confident and wears pretty things. The person that I plan to be is beautiful inside and out. She loves church and loves wearing dresses. Watch out world, you haven't seen the real me in years. The real me wants to be feminine and beautiful all the time.

Dear raincoat, I know that I have hidden under you for years now. It is time for me to blossom into a real person with something to say to the world around me. I have started thinking about what kind of job I want. I want to work in a recording studio, work around musicians and songs. I would like to work with famous singers on albums. I was born to write love songs and will prove it one day.

Today while I walked on the treadmill at the gym, I started to wonder as I saw my reflection in the mirror. How did I get to this point in my life? How did I get to the point of wanting to die? I mean sometimes suicidal thoughts cross my mind when I look at my fat body. It's time for me to change my outer self, to match my inside personality. The real me is fun and loves people. The real me loves romance and laughing all the time. That is the real me. For years now all I see when I look in the mirror is a tired-out mommy with ugly hair and clothes. I breathe life out and don't take it in so much that I forgot who I really was.

The universe was ready to help me. One day I developed an allergy to cheese, and then the next day, it was peanuts. My food allergies began to get out of control, leaving me no choices. I was eating very little. I started losing weight. I was left eating fruits and vegetables. I gave up milk products and peanut butter, the two things I found most enjoyable. My food addiction was taken away by allergies that started taking my breathing away. Some nights I was scared I would die after a meal. My air supply was being cut off just for eating pizza, macaroni and cheese, and many other foods. Ice cream became a scary choice to eat. My throat began to bother me a great deal.

Each day became harder and harder to breathe if I consumed most foods. I wondered if I would ever be the same person again. My clothes began to fall off of me. I knew I must be losing weight, but I didn't want to get on the scale for any reason. A doctor told me once that it's not the weight but the way you look that matters. He had a really good point about that.

I went to an allergist only to find I had no allergies at all, but it was a disorder with my lungs making me cough all the time after eating. Now a new goal was set into place, to run daily and regain strength in my lungs. My current weight is 189 pounds. I still have a long way to go to get to a healthy weight. The doctor told me that my bronchitis damaged my lungs and that I needed to rebuild them. I don't know a thing about jogging and running, but I will learn fast. I need to be stronger, and I need to be healthy. I can't eat much food, and I have no idea when I will feel well again.

When I eat most foods, my throat swells and makes me feel like I can't breathe. There is a fear that some foods are dangerous for me. I don't understand how cheese and all milk products have turned on me like an enemy. I am trying to find what I can consume that won't swell my throat. Peanut butter, my favorite food of all time, is swelling my throat. My family doctor says I must keep eating things I seem allergic to. She says that if I give them up completely, it makes it worse.

I am losing weight from this health situation, and it's not good. I feel weak, and I wonder if I will ever feel well enough to eat a whole meal. I am jogging, but I have very little air. I feel like I am drowning in my lungs from the inside out, some days. I haven't gotten on the scale, but I can tell I have lost quite a bit of weight. Is this how my prayers were answered? I developed a terrible eating allergy that takes my air and swells my throat. I have no idea if I will ever feel good again.

Moved to Florida

My husband took a job in Florida. It was a job transfer. He was happy about it, because he would be back near his sister. I honestly didn't know what to expect from a new state. I am used to Arkansas and tornadoes. We made it here, and it took me two weeks to adapt to my surroundings. My weight dropped from 189 to 180 while I ate very little and was busy unpacking. We moved to a rental house that is not what I am used to. I moved from a clean nice home. The rental has giant roaches, and they chase me. It's a different world here. I hate eating with roaches running by and lizards on my window.

When I open my door, there are lizards looking at things or hanging out. I worry that an alligator will attack me on my way to the mailbox. It's stupid for me to say that, since I don't live near water.

Everyone speaks Spanish everywhere I go. That worries me, since I know only English, and I am bad at that. Spanish is something I really must learn if I want a good job here. I started watching Spanish-speaking soap operas to learn Spanish. The only thing I am learning from these shows is that they are naughtier than English-speaking soaps.

It's now August 6, 2011, my current weight is 161. I sure have come a long way from 200 in April or 230 in January. I still have a very long way to go. I eat only once a day now. I exercise with Tae Bo one hour daily. I exercise even when I do not want to. I get on the scale and can't believe that I have come so far.

I still hate my size. I look in the mirror, and I see my clothes are falling off me, but I hate myself for not being ninety pounds yet. I have to lose seventy-one pounds to get to my goal. I imagine that I will have lots of hungry days with over exercising in them.

I decided to audition for a music show, the new show where you sing and they have their backs to you. I am sick and have no singing voice today. I have six days to get well. I'm praying it will happen. I need to take this opportunity to audition, since it's in Orlando, only twenty minutes away. I am going to sing an R&B song. I can't wait. This audition was a great motivator for me to lose weight. I lost ten pounds the last two weeks, just dreaming of getting on the show. I will give it my all and hope they choose me for the show. If not, then I am thankful for the additional weight loss that happened to me.

Me Now

I am in reality now. I no longer dream about true love. I must have read one too many romance novels or watched too many romantic made-for-TV shows. What I want is to be thankful for everything I have now and stop complaining so much in my head about what I don't have. So what if my clothes look like I live on the streets? This is nothing to me now. I want to focus on losing more weight and becoming the person I need to be here on earth. I haven't smiled much since going off the meds. Anti-depression meds are the only way I can smile. It's not my fault. I am a very different person off meds or on them.

Anti-depression medication has always made me a more pleasant person, but the headaches I got were horrible. I love being headache free now, but I have been missing laughing and smiling.

I've been online a lot lately, praying for people. Some call me a prayer warrior. Most have no idea that I am so lonely or unhappy in my real life. It's easier to hide your true self-online. No one would want to know what life is really like for me.

I don't have a date for when I will make my weight goal. I have decided to be good to myself and stop trying to be so unforgiving about weight-loss time. I am doing great and no longer weigh 230. Some would be surprised to have seen me that size. Once they see the smaller me, they won't remember my highest weight. My clothes no longer fit me, and I need smaller ones. There is no use to run out to the store, though, because I plan to keep going and going with the weight loss.

I am looking at life with a real sense of who I am now. I know that if I want things to happen, I have to make them happen. I am in control of my life now, and I plan to turn things around. Never do I want to feel afraid again. I am well educated and plan to find a great job in the future. I believe that a year from now, I will be living a completely different life than the one I see now.

Goodwill Store

I had to find a dress for choir Christmas performance, so I went to Goodwill. There was a dress there that looked like one for a princess. It was a size eight, and I am a size fourteen. I wanted to buy it, but deep down, I knew my large chest would never fit into it. I showed the dress to Chris. He was hesitant for me to spend ten dollars on a dress I couldn't zip.

I bought the dress and took it home. I tried to put it on. It didn't fit the way I wanted it to. I decided to start running to lose weight. The first day, I ran three miles. The next day, I ran four miles. By day four, I was at six miles. There is something really great about running. It makes me feel good. My weight is currently 156, and I am feeling like I have my whole life ahead of me to smile. I am going to smile more than I ever did. Right now I am closer to not being obese. I use exercise tapes daily and find that exercise is a great reducer of anxiety.

When I see skinny people, I often wonder if they too suffered from obesity like me. Did they come back from being super fat to being smaller? I look in the mirror at this point, and I am still feeling that I have so much to lose. Tomorrow I will exercise more, and I will try harder to be confident in my own accomplishments. This week I have one goal, to get under 150. I will push myself to do better and exercise more hours each day. One day really soon, no one will remember I was ever fat.

I am in dire need of a fat friend, someone who could talk to me daily and share her fears and goals. All I have is me, and that isn't enough. I pray to God one day that I live near someone kind who will share thoughts with me. I need friends who care about me. I need anyone who will give me a moment of her time. It's a closed world, not having family around and no friends to laugh with.

This weight makes me angry when I go to the doctor. I get on the scale and the skinny nurse looks at me like she is shocked the scale goes that high. Yes, I have a giant booty. I don't feel good about it, world.

I need to motivate myself in 2012 to be lean. I promise myself that I will lose all the weight I planned to lose. Food will no longer control me on a depression day or a bad day. My heart and soul need to be healed, and that won't happen until I am in shape and feeling well again.

When I look in the mirror I wonder if I will ever wear clothes that pretty people wear. I want to be thin and feel beautiful. No man has ever really treated me like I was beautiful. They act like I am ugly and not worth knowing. Can't anyone see that I feel more than the words that come out of their mouths? It's what people don't say that hurts the most. When people don't compliment you after you send a pretty photo, you know they think you're fat or ugly. Silence is a dead ringer for a lack of attraction for you.

January 2012

I wonder how another year could have passed by. I weighed in at 156 after coming home from the in-laws' house. I wasn't good on my diet while staying with them. I wanted to be. I will start jogging thirty minutes a day, six days a week to try to lose the weight I gained to begin with.

Falling off the diet wagon is something my husband often fears for me. He tries to hide candy and other things that send me into a frenzy of depression.

The pressure to lose the weight has taken a toll on me. I fear that I will never get to my goals. Migraines are happening more and more, and I rarely sleep. I even started taking diuretics and diet pills. The diet pills make me act weird. I feel like hitting people while on them. They overwhelm me sometimes with the energy they give me. I hate diet pills, but don't know how to get over the plateau that is trapping my body.

Now it is the end of the month, and I am amazingly feeling that my body is starting to get smaller and smaller. My weight is 144 and my size sixteen and fourteen pants are falling off me. It is a true dream of mine to be skinny. I went to the store and put on a shirt that was an 8/10, and it fit me. How happy I am!

I still can't smile yet, though. I have a long way to go before I get to ninety pounds. My husband told me last night I am not hot yet and need to lose more weight, and it hurt my feelings, but he was right. I have a long way to go to be beautiful.

Every day now, I run an hour and do exercises. I am physically tired from all the exercise. The weight stays on, but my body is reshaping itself. My size twelve pants that I got for Christmas are baggy now.

My soul cries out for someone to hug me, tell me I am doing good, but there is no one calling me or talking to me daily. I have to lean on myself.

My children fight all the time and rarely speak to me. It's a lonely world I live in and my battle to fight. I have absolutely no clothes to wear now and no money to go to the store to get clothes. I wish I had money, but I have no money to buy clothes. I feel sad about this fact, but feel in my heart I will win the lottery and be rich this year. I know that statement sounds wild, but I plan to be rich by June. I can then afford clothes for the kids and me.

Some women would love to be in size twelve and be smaller than they are. My weight is keeping me from being truly loved and respected, and I hate it. It's my enemy.

I had a friend text that I had low self-esteem and needed help. It was a horrible thing to say to me, because it made me feel even worse, by pointing out my flaws. I am full of pain within my heart over my own eating and my own slowness in getting my body in shape. I am new today. No one can touch me; my heart is not going to give up, not again.

February's Girl

Guess what. Today is February 4. I now weigh in at 140. I did weigh that this morning. I shouldn't have obsessed and weighed myself this late at night to make sure I was still at the amount.

Raincoat, I haven't seen you in months. I bet you would not fit me anymore. I want to wear you again, because you remind me of how far I have come. A few days ago, I tried on a bathing suit that was an 8-10, and it fit. Feelings of pure joy raced through my mind. I looked in the mirror wondering how someone like me finally got to this size. It was me, and I looked pretty. I never felt that way before.

I wanted to cry, but I waited until later, while running for an hour, to let the happiness hit me.

I realized something, now that I am not as big as I was. I realized that happiness comes from many places. I find that even with weight loss, things are bothering me. I am weighted down mentally by people I need to be close to who won't give me the time of day. Reality is that you can't control others' emotions or the way they treat you. All you can do is pinpoint exactly what makes you happy. I am on my way to feeling better than I ever did before. I made my husband take photos of me today. I told him that in a week I would weigh in the 130s, not the 140s.

I believe I can do anything I set my mind to now. The only thing stopping me from being fantastically successful, is me. Self-doubt does a number on me and probably a big portion of the world. I have made the mistake of sharing some of my weaknesses with friends. I am ready to live as if I have no weaknesses now.

Right here in my world lives dreams that I will find. I will make my own destiny from this day forward. When I look in the mirror I see that I am a child of God. I don't need anyone to say I am perfect or hot or anything else. The me I needed most was the one who loves herself. I do now understand the meaning of self-esteem. Every little insult and every relationship that tore me down built inside me a self-hate I no longer have. I know that insecure people always bring those around them down to hide who they really are. From this day forward, I won't chase friends who don't want to e-mail or call or know me. I don't need them anymore. I am far better off alone than with people who don't accept me for who I am. I have spent a lifetime being there for others. It's time I be there for myself. Learning to be good to me is very important. With weight loss, I can now focus on being stronger as a woman. I know I am a good mom. I want all aspects of my life to shine like the light I have inside my soul.

What I want for me is better choices regarding how I spend my time. Time is very easy to waste. I had my husband take a photo of me today to make a comparison between when I was a size 28 and one at size 10-12. I didn't look the same. I felt a sickness come over me, looking at the "before" picture. I didn't know I was that big. I am sad that I couldn't see how large I was. Weight creeps up on you every year, and it begins to be normal, so you don't notice it the way others do.

My heart sees now how important fitness is. I work out daily now. I find that even the smallest things make me smile. I run an hour a day, and it keeps my weight off. I started to shrink my body when I started to run. I don't want to forget how hard it was to get to where I am now.

June 2012

Here I am ready to see family. I know they will be shocked at my new size. I used to be someone they were ashamed of. I could tell that I made people uncomfortable when I sat on benches that bent. I will be visiting my siblings and Dad in a little while. I now weigh 120 pounds and have lost a great deal of weight since they saw me at Christmastime. I am a size six now, and my jeans are baggy.

I feel a sense of shyness for some reason. I don't know how people will see me when I get to my hometown.

My sister says I look ill. She is not used to me looking this small. I have been in town a few days now and can tell that people are surprised I lost the weight. I was fat my entire life.

I plan to go home and lose even more weight. Although I have lost a great amount of weight, I still need to lose more for my tiny bone structure and height. I am only four feet, eleven inches, and some people don't realize what the healthy weight for someone my height is.

As I spend time with family, I feel like everyone is looking at me weirdly. They keep asking me to eat. I guess I look hungry.

Food no longer has a hold of me. I eat but don't focus on it anymore. I used to live to eat. My life revolved around what I snacked on, and I could eat a whole bag of candy bars. I would become ill now, if

I overate like that. I am no longer the same person I started out to be.

We left town from our family visit, and I had not gained weight. I was happy about that. Sometimes when I travel, fast food can take me in a backwards direction, weight gain. This time around, I packed healthy things in the car and didn't eat much on the road. I knew I had no way to burn the calories.

Do I worry about eating sugar or soft drinks now? No. In fact I actually drink one soda a day to keep from having a migraine. What I realized is that the last meal of the day is one I must watch carefully. Never eat more than you intend to burn off.

I love visiting family. I am glad that I got this chance to go to see them. I cherish my parents, my siblings, my sister-in-law, and my nieces and nephews. I know that life is very precious, so I won't ever forget my time in North Carolina this summer. My kids were happy to see their grandpa again. I was pleased to notice my dad was watching some shows I liked. We both love stuff on the History Channel.

As I get older I realize how much family means and how time with them makes me happy. Losing all this weight is really about being around and being healthy for my children. I want to be there a lifetime for them. Being the right weight is a very positive thing. My son even runs with me, some days. This summer he decided to get in to shape with me. Losing weight was a good thing to show my children that you can make changes and put forth the effort to be better.

I just registered for graduate school and feel glad about that. I believe in myself as a Christian. I want to be the best parent and person I can be. I want to excel at anything I try to do.

Weight loss is a journey many will take, and I am here to say you can improve your life. Never give up on your goals when it comes to your health.

The Final Chapter

I have transformed into someone else on this journey. Today is Sept 6, 2012. The new person I am doesn't need validation or love, like the person I was, before. What I actually thirsted for was peace. I needed peace in my soul to let go of pain I had deeply held onto for a lifetime.

I am at peace with my body and my life now. Every choice I make from now on is my own to make. If I fall, then I will get back up. What have I learned in my journey to be smaller? I am responsible for every bite of food that goes in my mouth. For better health, I need to control every emotion that causes me stress. Stress brings weight on fast and is difficult for me to lose. I am a stress eater.

I find my raincoat is no longer needed to hide me. I am ready to step out in whatever clothes I have on. The world can see me now. I am walking without a crutch. My current weight is 110, and I am a size four. My crutch was my daily raincoat. It hid my fat and hid my pain. Now I am a changed person.

My journey to where I am now took place like everyone else's journey who is obese. I was at a weak point in my life and had to make a change or die sooner than I was supposed to. How do I explain to you how far I have come? If it were miles that I walked, then I would have reached another country. All I know now is that my weight will go down more and more. I will help others find happiness through fitness and eating right. I want to be a friend and support those who have no idea how much they can accomplish. I will motivate others to change their bodies, because I know how hard it can be.

Within me exists greatness that I never knew before. I am stronger, more loving, and healthy now. I praise God for being by my side the entire time. He never left my side, and I am forever grateful for that.

Finding happiness and breathing life is important, so make sure you do that. Life is a dance, so don't waste time sitting on the sideline like I did. Hide from no one, but keep your spirit lit up to face each day. Exercise every single day, if you want to see weight loss. I believe everyone has the potential to be strong. Find your greatness now.

If I could go back in time, I would try hard to love more and live more, but I have the future ahead of me, and so do you. If you have weight to lose, start now. The best you is yet to come.

I know from my own years of struggling that greatness is within, and you have to find strength, even when you have nothing. "I will be thin and healthy." I said it over and over in my head; now I live it.

Weight can be lost; just believe in yourself. You can do anything. This is what I believe.

Here I am weighing in at 230, barely fitting in the chair.

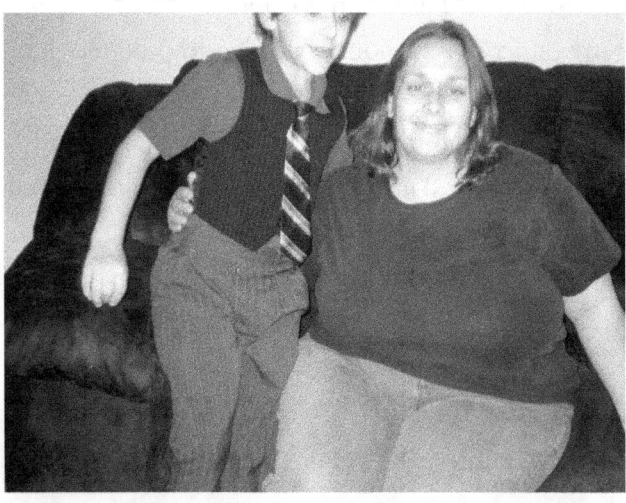

This is my son Luke with me. I was ashamed to have my photo taken, being so obese. Luke was ashamed of me too, and it made him sad.

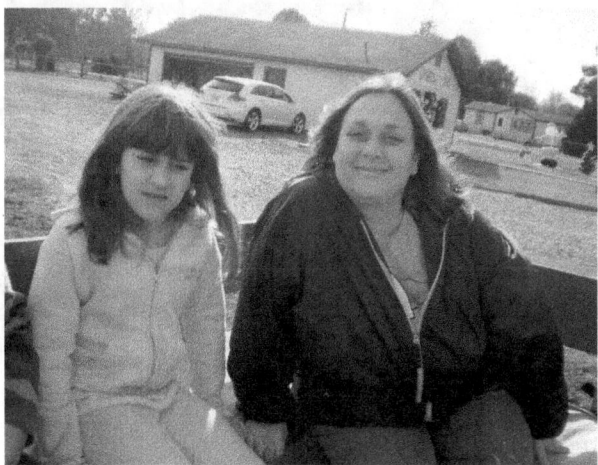

This was me in my raincoat, hiding fat, December 2010. Hannah is beside me.

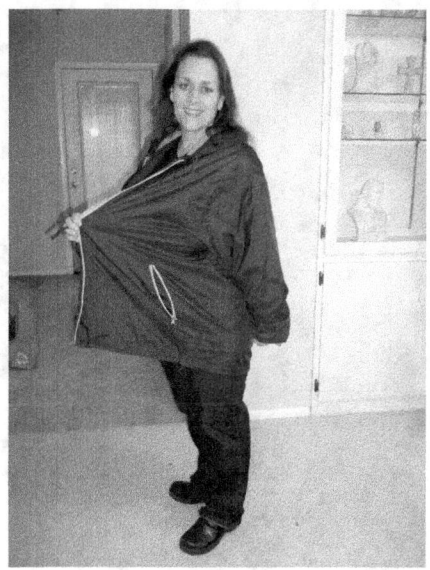

Here I am in my raincoat. It's now too big for me to wear. I am ready to start my new life without it. The next time I wear a raincoat, it will actually be raining outside, and the color will be very pretty. I changed inside and out.

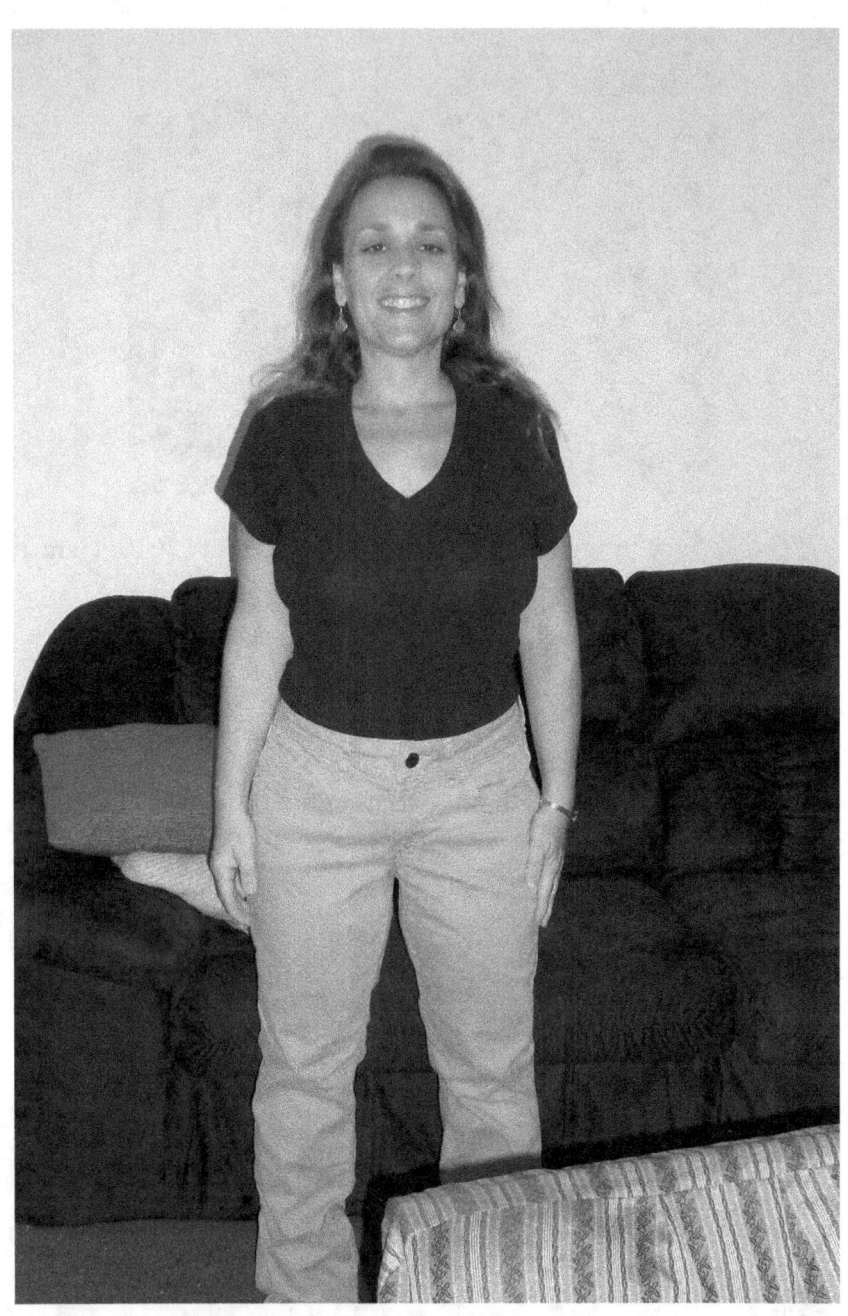

Here I am size four, happy, and healthy.

www.ingramcontent.com/pod-product-compliance
Lightning Source LLC
Chambersburg PA
CBHW070030300526
45794CB00001B/444